Localization of Skin Lesions in Images Using the U-Net Architecture

AF720496

Masaru

Localization of Skin Lesions in Images Using the U-Net Architecture

First Edition June 2025

Copyright © 2025 Masaru

Written by Masaru

TABLE OF CONTENTS

CHAPTER NO.	TITLE	PAGE NO.

CHAPTER NO.	TITLE	PAGE NO.

CHAPTER NO.	TITLE	PAGE NO.

CHAPTER NO.	TITLE	PAGE NO.

CHAPTER 1

INTRODUCTION

1.1 BACKGROUND

Psoriasis is an inflammatory chronic skin disorder that affects 2%–3% of the global population including 1%–5% of children (Parisi & Symmons 2013). According to Cameron and Voohees (2014) and Perera *et al.* (2012), psoriasis is a bimodal illness that has a large onset around age 20–30 and a subsequent, lower peak onset around age 50–60. Although the precise cause of psoriasis is still unknown, a number of important factors are thought to be involved, including immune system dysfunction, environmental triggers, disturbance of the skin barrier, and genetic vulnerability (Raychaudhuri *et al.* 2014). Psoriasis has five major categories: guttate, pustular, inverse, vulgaris (plaque), and erythrodermic. Plaque psoriasis accounts for around 85% to 90% of cases of psoriasis, making it the most common type (Griffiths & Barker 2007).

In the majority of cases, psoriasis causes severe physical and psychological suffering and disability, which negatively impacts the quality of life of the patient. Psoriasis sufferers frequently experience feelings of shame and guilt, and the condition stigmatises them (Hrehorow *et al.* 2012). Psoriasis has been observed to have an influence on patients' interpersonal connections, as well as their sexual well-being and ability for intimacy (de Korte *et al.* 2004, Kimball *et al.* 2005). Psoriasis has a detrimental social impact at work, which might show up as prejudice and make it harder to get a work. In the year prior, nearly 60% of psoriasis patients who were also employed reported missing work because of their condition. Many Americans lose their lives to issues related to psoriasis each year (Pearce *et al.* 2006). Physical co morbidities associated with psoriasis can shorten life expectancy as a result of its adverse effects. There are many diseases associated with psoriatic arthritis, including metabolic syndrome, diabetes, obesity, inflammatory bowel disease (IBD), and cardiovascular disease (CVD) (Love and others 2011; Kimball and others 2008; Armstrong and others 2013; Gelfand & Yeung 2012).

1.2 THE HUMAN SKIN PHYSIOLOGY

The human body's most significant sensory organ is the skin. It takes up roughly 20 square feet. In addition to controlling body temperature and providing touch, heat, and cold sensibility, the skin shields us from microbes and the outside world.

Skin has three layers as shown in Figure 1.1.

- A person's skin tone is determined by their epidermis, which serves as a waterproof barrier and determines their complexion.
- Under the epidermis, the dermis consists of hair follicles, sweat glands, and an extensive network of connective tissues.
- A deeper layer of subcutaneous tissue, known as the hypodermis, consists of connective tissue and fat. Skin is coloured by the pigment melanin, which is produced by special cells called melanocytes. Melanocytes are present in the skin's outermost layer.

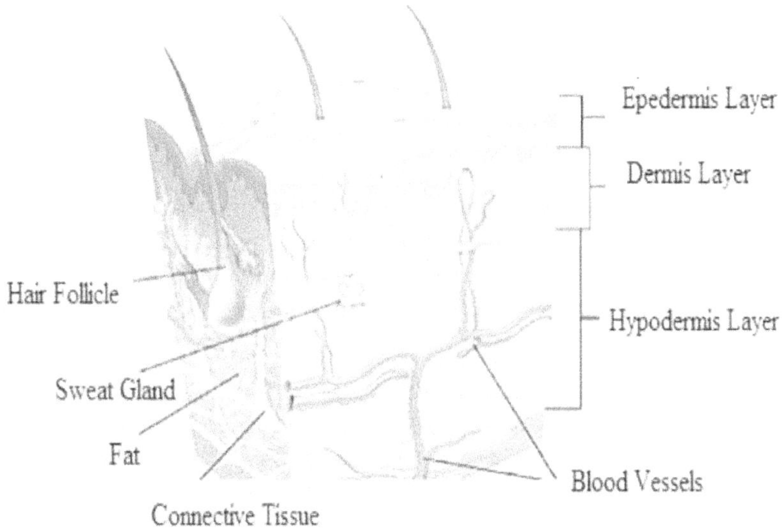

Figure 1.1 Anatomy of the skin, showing the epidermis, the dermis, and subcutaneous (hypodermis) tissue

1.2.1 Types of Skin Lesions

Seven types skin disease are classified as follows;

- Melanoma: The worst type of skin cancer, melanoma is caused by sun exposure and other reasons. A skin biopsy can be used to diagnose melanoma.
- Basal cell carcinoma: The kind of skin cancer that is most common. Because it grows and spreads more slowly than melanoma, basal cell carcinoma is less harmful.
- Seborrheic keratosis: A benign growth that resembles a "stuck-on" wart and is frequently irritating. If seborrheic keratoses are uncomfortable, a doctor can remove them.
- Actinic keratosis: An exposed skin lesion that appears crusty or scaly. Actinic keratoses can sometimes progress to cancer. Squamous cell carcinoma: This type of skin cancer is frequently diagnosed as an ulcer or an abnormal growth that is difficult to heal. It typically appears in sun-exposed regions.

- Eczema: Dermatitis, or skin irritation, resulting in an itchy rash. The most common cause is an overactive immune system.
- Psoriasis: An autoimmune disease that causes a variety of skin rashes. The most typical kind of psoriasis is characterised by silvery, scaly skin lesions.

1.3 TYPES OF SKIN DISEASES

Skin conditions are a widespread ailment that impact millions of individuals globally. Comprehending these illnesses is essential, since they can greatly affect an individual's standard of living. Numerous broad categories, such as infectious, autoimmune, genetic, and environmental, can be used to group skin diseases. Infectious skin diseases are caused by bacteria, viruses, fungi, or parasites and include conditions such as acne, warts, and ringworm. Autoimmune skin diseases occur when the immune system attacks healthy skin cells and can result in conditions such as psoriasis and lupus. Genetic skin diseases are inherited and include disorders such as albinism and ichthyosis. By understanding the different types of skin diseases, healthcare professionals can better diagnose and treat patients with these conditions.

Infectious Skin Diseases

- Bacterial skin infections (e.g. cellulitis, impetigo)
- Viral skin infections (e.g. herpes, warts)
- Fungal skin infections (e.g. ringworm, athlete's foot)

Non -Infectious Skin Diseases

- Autoimmune skin diseases (e.g. psoriasis, lupus)
- Genetic skin diseases (e.g. epidermolysis bullosa,albinism)
- Skin cancer (e.g. melanoma, basal cell carcinoma)

1.4 AUTOIMMUNE SKIN DISEASES (E.G. PSORIASIS, LUPUS)

Skin cancer (e.g. melanoma, basal cell carcinoma) - Genetic skin disorders (e.g. albinism, epidermolysis bullosa) - Allergic skin reactions (e.g. eczema, hives) - Inflammatory skin conditions (e.g. rosacea, acne) - Pigmentary disorders (e.g. vitiligo, melasma). Proper diagnosis and treatment of these skin diseases are crucial to prevent complications and improve the quality of life for patients. Healthcare professionals should be knowledgeable about the different types of skin diseases and their symptoms to provide accurate diagnoses and effective treatments. In addition to medical interventions, lifestyle changes such as maintaining good hygiene and avoiding triggers can also help manage certain skin conditions. It is important for patients to seek medical attention promptly if they notice any changes in their skin or experience persistent symptoms. With proper care and management, many skin diseases can be controlled or even cured, allowing patients to lead healthy and fulfilling lives.

1.5 PATHOGENESIS OF PSORIASIS

Prior to investigating the pathological alterations that occur to place in psoriatic skin, it is critical to realise the typical process of keratinocyte transformation and maturation. In normal human skin, the epidermis' lowest layer contains the dividing cells, or epidermal stem cells. These cells proliferate at random to create new stem cells or transit amplifying cells. They commit to differentiation after a specific level of cell proliferation. The epidermal differentiation unit is made up of epidermal stem cells and their differentiated offspring cells. Every stage of differentiation is regulated by distinct markers, including filagrin, caspase 14, loricirin, involucrin, keratin 1, 5, 10, 14, and others. The cells move suprabasally and differentiate into stratum spinosum, grnulosum, lucidium, and ultimately stratum corneum cells (corneocytes), depending on the differentiation markers exhibited. Corneocytes are terminally differentiated, anuclear keratnocytes devoid of extra cytoplasm. This layer of epidermis is continuously renewed by desquamation since corneocytes make up the stratum corneum. In the case of normal skin, it takes 28 days to entirely regenerate the epidermis (Coondoo 2012, El-Darouti & Hay 2010, Raychaudhuri *et al.* 2014).

In psoriatic skin, there is a decrease in the time required for epidermal replacement (also known as the epidermal transit time), an increase in the turnover of epidermal cells, and an inability of the cells to finish differentiating. Consequently, the skin displays erythomatous, scaly sores. The epidermis extends to the dermis as extended rete ridges in psoriatic skin, exhibiting considerable epidermal thickening (acanthosis) and abnormal epidermal cell differentiation (parakerototic). Psoriasis is caused by aberrant proliferation of keratinocytes with inadequate differentiation; the redness of psoriatic skin lesions is caused by significant dilatation of blood vessels in the dermal papillae. As one of the major characteristics of psoriatic skin, the dermis and epidermis are deeply infiltrated with immune and inflammatory cells (Godin & Touitou 2007, Randal Wickett & Marty Visscher 2006). A single anomaly in the proliferation and differentiation of a particular type of cell type cannot explain psoriasis as a disease caused by an aberrant generation of an inflammatory cytokine. This disease is the result of a number of interrelated variables working together with a favorable genetic background and the appropriate environmental conditions.

Psoriasis and altered immunity: Previously, psoriasis was thought to be a skin disease caused by aberrant keratinocytes; Overactive immune systems have now been identified as the cause of the condition. (Nedoszytko *et al.* 2014, Traub & Marshall 2007). The pathogenesis of psoriasis can be split into three steps: early activation of T cells, subsequent migration into the skin, and cytokine production by T cells, as shown in Figure 1.2 (Jadali *et al.* 2007).

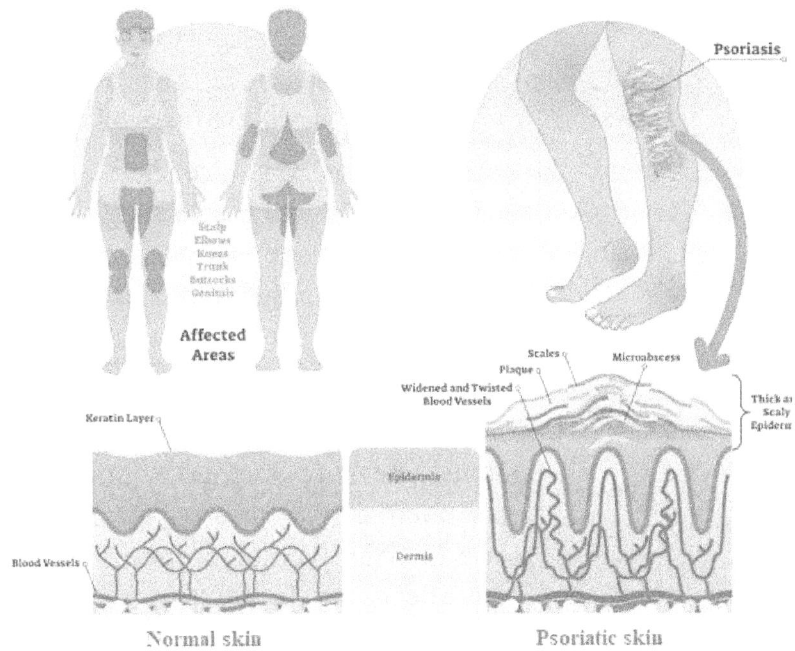

Figure 1.2 The structural changes in the skin under the influence of psoriasis

1.6 TYPES OF PSORIASIS

According to the appearance and location of the lesions, psoriasis is divided into many types (Preeti K Suresh *et al.* 2013).

Table 1.1 Types of psoriasis

Sl No.	Types	Features
1	Plaque	This is the most prevalent type of psoriasis, where red areas coated with a deposit of dead skin cells because the skin to look as elevated silvery white scales. The condition typically affects the elbow, lower back, scalp, and knees.
2	Pustular	Adults are the primary patients of this type of illness. It could be universal or restricted to specific bodily parts, such the hands and feet. It usually progresses in a cycle of skin reddening, pustule development, and scaling.

Table 1.1 (Continued)

Sl No.	Types	Features
3	Guttate	Red spots on the skin characterize this type of skin condition, commonly affecting the trunk, limbs, face, ears, and occasionally the scalp. This particular ailment may occur before or alongside other types of psoriasis, including plaque psoriasis.
4	Inverse	Lesions in this case predominantly manifest in the skin folds of the body, including the genitals, armpits, under the breasts, or buttocks. These skin folds, referred to as flexures, are also termed flexural psoriasis. This type of psoriasis is notably painful and challenging.
5	Erythrodermic	This type of psoriasis is the least common, affecting approximately 1 to 2 percent of people at some point in their lives. It usually shows up in those who have unstable plaque psoriasis. Skin exfoliation and extensive burning redness are characteristics of this type.
6	Nail	Psoriasis affects the nails of the fingers and toenails, resulting in pitted, thick fingernails with ridges which elevate the nail and give it an uneven shape.
7	Scalp	The scaly plaque-like lesions on this scalp have a well-defined boundary. The illness is typified by a severe case of hyperkeratosis that is closely surrounded with hairs. Although it doesn't happen often, heavy traction applied to the hair might cause permanent hair loss.

1.7 SKIN PHENOTYPE AND HISTOLOGY OF PSORIASIS

Psoriasis most commonly manifests as plaques. In addition to the scalp, knees, elbows, and lumbar area, the plaques are red, scaly, well-defined, silvery-white, and dry. Patients often report excruciating itching from the erythematous, usually symmetrical plaques. Psoriasis Area and Severity Index (PASI) and Physician's Global Evaluation (PGA) are two methods for estimating plaque severity. In addition to erythema, induration, desquamation, and body surface area, the PASI scale measures area and intensity. PGA was developed as a substitute assessment metric due to the complexity of the PASI calculation. An analysis of the PGA is used to determine whether the severity of a lesion is constant or fluctuating. It is interesting to note that in patients with chronic plaque psoriasis, normal skin appears adjacent to the psoriatic plaques. In recent years, a number of studies have demonstrated that uninvolved tissues contain a unique collection of genes that, when activated, can explain why uninvolved tissues become involved. It is improbable to isolate a single triggering mechanism, nonetheless, considering the variety of cell types involved inthis conversion (Figure 1.3).

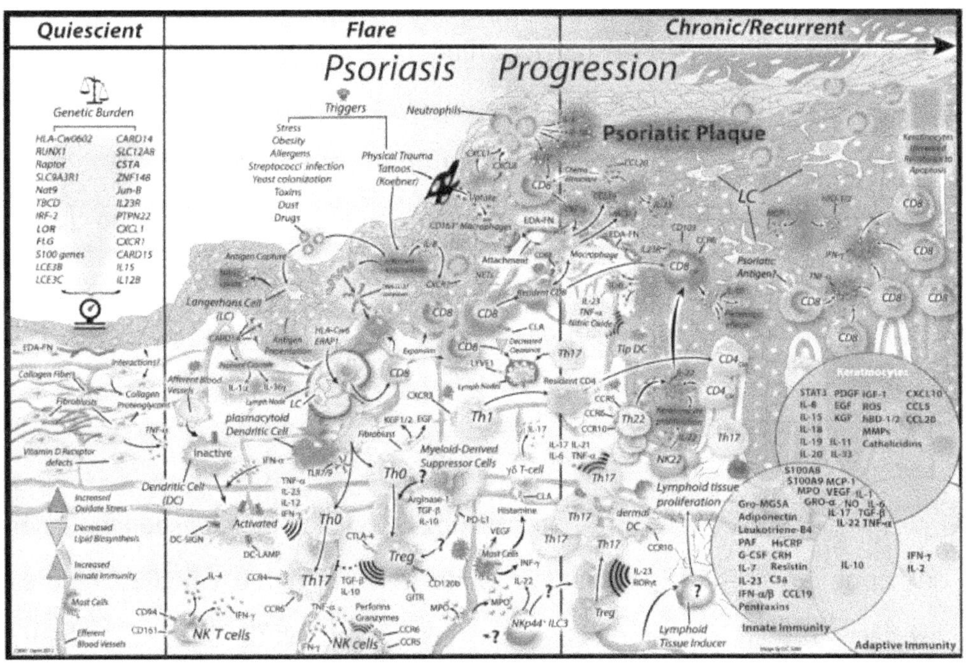

Figure 1.3 Key signal in psoriasis development

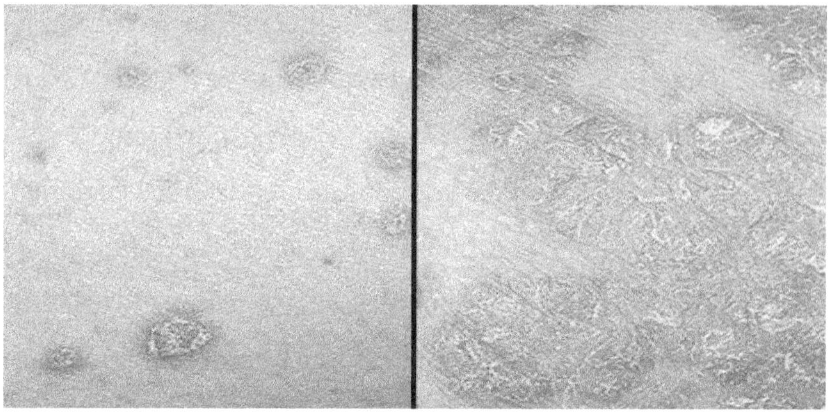

Figure 1.4 Psoriasis in Human Skin

1.8 POTENTIAL CAUSES/TRIGGERS OF PSORIASIS

a) Genes

Psoriasis patients have a variety of gene variants linked to immunological and skin barrier function, according to genetic studies. Psoriasis incidence analyses showed that there is a 70% chance that monozygotic twins will have the condition, compared to a 20% chance for dizygotic twins. According to pedigree studies, children who have one affected parent or both affected parents have a 20% and 65% probability, respectively, of acquiring psoriasis.

b) PSORS1

PSORS1 on chromosome 6p21 was the first associated psoriasis susceptibility (PSORS) locus. Although it is debatable whether gene causes psoriasis, research has indicated that this region has the biggest influence on the heredity of the condition. It is generally believed that the HLA-C gene is most likely the gene responsible for the PSORS1 gene in the major histocompatibility complex class 1 area.

c) PSORS2/CARD14 mutation

PSORS2 was located on chromosome 17q25 by means of family association mapping and genome-wide linkage scanning. The discovery of a gain-of-function mutation in CARD14 on this locus has been attributed to next-generation sequencing of patients with familial psoriasis. Furthermore, several missense mutations in CARD14 were found in psoriatic individuals as well as 2.7-fold higher levels of CARD14 mRNA. Increased NF-kβ activation in the presence of CARD14 mutations can lead to psoriasis by up regulating the expression of key psoriatic chemokines such CCL20, CXCL8/IL-8, and IL-36γ/IL-1F9.20. The psoriatic cascade may also be activated by another environmental factor (Figure 1.1).

1.9 RISK FACTORS FOR PSORIASIS

Psoriasis cannot be attributed to a single reason; instead, it appears to be the result of several genetic variables interacting with advantageous environmental circumstances (Jadali *et al.* 2007).

Genetics: It has been noted that 30% of psoriatic cases have a family history including a first- or second-degree relative. There have been reports of nine chromosomal susceptibility loci (PSORS 1-9) expressing abnormally. Polymorphisms in genes that regulate inflammation and angiogenesis have been linked to PSORS (Jadali *et al.* 2007).

Trauma: One well-known cause of psoriasis is injury to the dermal papilla. Inflammatory plaque psoriasis can result from injuries of any kind, including chemical and physical trauma, surgical wounds, and some bacterial infections. The Koebner phenomenon is the mechanism by which an injury causes psoriasis to develop. Koebner phenomenon's precise mechanism is unknown (Divya *et al.* 2016, Jadali *et al.* 2007).

Infections: A few weeks following streptococcal throat infections, there have been examples of documented guttate psoriasis. Whether there is a connection between these two is unclear (Jadali *et al.* 2007).

Sun light: Even while most psoriatic patients believe that sunlight is good, there are reports that intense sunlight may actually make the illness worse in certain circumstances (Jadali *et al.* 2007).

Smoking: One significant risk factor for long-term plaque psoriasis is smoking. After smoking, nicotine buildup can affect the immune system's ability to respond both innately and adaptively. It has the ability to control how immune cells behave and how much proinflammatory cytokines they release. In addition to increasing calcium influx in keratinocytes, nicotinic cholinergic receptors also play a critical role in adhesion, differentiation, and upward migration of keratinocytes.

Alcohol intake: Children with psoriasis who consume alcohol are at an increased risk for developing the disease. Increasing histamine release is one of the mechanisms by which alcohol exacerbates skin sores. Alcohol consumption is associated with excessive consumption of fats and a lack of consumption of fruits and vegetables.

Hormones: Hormone fluctuations cause variations in the psoriatic condition. A flare-up of the disease may happen during the postpartum time, but it is reported that pregnant conditions improve the disease, which may have started at adolescence. Immune cells have receptors on their surface or within of them that allow sex hormones to interact with them. According to Jadali *et al.* (2007), steroid hormones have the ability to control the generation of antibodies and the growth of immune cells.

Drugs: A flare-up of an illness can be brought on by some medications, such as benzodiazepines, organic nitrates, beta blockers, lithium salts, non-steroidal anti-inflammatory medicines, angiotensin converting enzyme inhibitors, antimalarials, and stopping systemic corticosteroids.

Diet: A low-calorie diet can enhance the clinical state of psoriasis by reducing the formation of leukotriene B4 (LT-B4) as a result of consuming less arachidonic acid. A diet high in vegetables and low in arachidonic acid is advantageous. Psoriasis is largely caused by oxidative stress, which is characterised by increased lipid peroxidation and decreased antioxidant enzyme activity. It is advised to have a diet high in antioxidants such flavonoids, carotenoids, and vitamin C as well as omega-3 fatty acids to lessen oxidative stress. Supplementing with vitamin D and vitamin B12 has been proven to be beneficial since cobalamin is necessary for the production of nucleic acids and vitamin D inhibits keratinocyte proliferation and accelerates its differentiation (Traub & Marshall 2007, Jadali *et al.* 2007).

Till date, it is accepted that psoriasis is a non curable but treatable disease. During the last few decades, many clinical and experimental researchers have done lots of work to improve the treatment policy of psoriasis. In order to control the inflammation caused by psoriasis, they have recommended various therapeutic agents, such as salicylic acid, steroid-based creams, coal-tar ointments and shampoos, phototherapy, methotrexate and biologics.

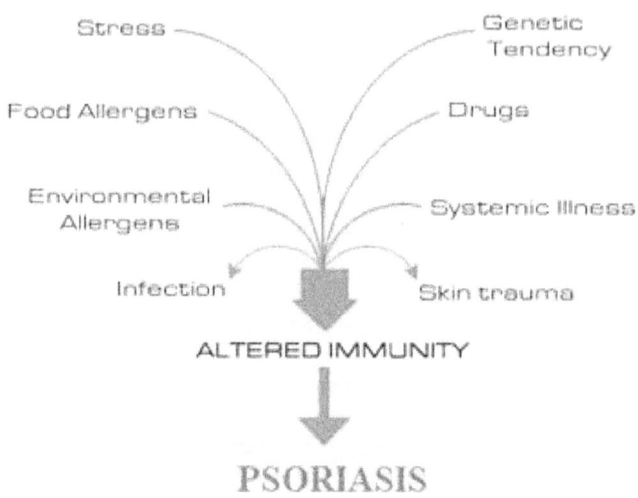

Figure 1.5 Various causative factors could influence the development of psoriasis

1.10 IMPORTANCE OF IMAGE SEGMENTATION AND CLASSIFICATION IN DIAGNOSIS AND TREATMENT

Psoriasis is a long-term autoimmune skin condition which leads to red, scaly patches to form on the body in different places. Image segmentation and classification are essential tools in the diagnosis and treatment of psoriasis. Accurate identification of psoriasis lesions can help doctors determine the severity of the disease and choose appropriate treatment options. By segmenting and classifying images of psoriasis lesions, doctors can also monitor changes in the condition over time and evaluate the effectiveness of different treatments. This makes image segmentation and classification crucial in improving patient outcomes and quality of life.

1.11 MEDICAL IMAGING

The term "medical imaging" describes the methods and procedures used to produce images of the human body for a range of therapeutic uses, including diagnosis, treatment, and the study of normal anatomy and function.

Diagnostic imaging is a vital tool in medicine. Among the imaging techniques that can map a subject's anatomy without requiring invasive procedures include digital mammography (MM), Computer Tomography (CT), Magnetic Resonance Imaging (MRI), and others. In the diagnosis of melanoma and other pigmented skin lesions one of the major imaging modalities used is dermoscopy. Over the past 20 years, numerous attempts have been made to enhance the clinical diagnosis of melanoma using the non-invasive dermoscopy technique. This technique allows for a clear and magnified visualisation of the skin's morphological structures that are invisible to the unaided eye.

Since these technologies have significantly expanded our understanding of both normal and diseased anatomy for medical research, they are an essential part of diagnostic and treatment planning. The size and volume of these medical images are increasing, making computer use necessary to aid in processing and analysis. Medical personnel must process a big quantity of images with significantly greater detail in the interim. For this kind of work, segmentation is typically an essential stage. Manual segmentation takes a long time, and the findings could not be repeatable or show intra- and inter-observer variability. For this reason, computer-aided segmentation is required to support medical staff in conducting effective and efficient analysis.

In order to help and automate some radiological procedures for the identification of anatomical structures and other areas of interest, computer algorithms are becoming more and more crucial. These techniques, known as image segmentation algorithms, are essential to many biomedical imaging applications, including treatment planning, computer-integrated surgery, pathology detection and localization, tissue volume quantification, anatomical structure investigation, and treatment planning. With the speed at which computer technology is developing, computer-aided image segmentation is becoming increasingly important for addressing problems in various image processing and computer vision domains.

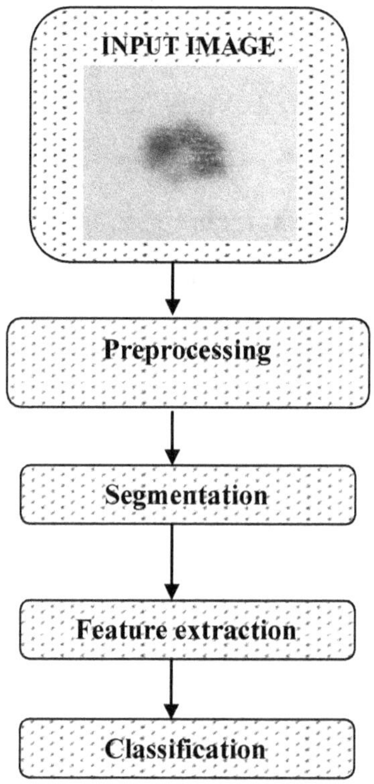

Figure 1.6 Flow chart of skin disease detection and classification

Image processing is a subset of signal processing in which the input is an image. A collection of parameters or qualities related to a picture can also be the outcome of image processing. During the segmentation process, a digital image is divided into several sections for convenient examination, changing the representation of the image. Segmenting an image is a technique used for identifying items and boundaries. For the purpose of segmenting images, numerous general-purpose algorithms and methods have been developed. Since there is no generic solution to the challenges involved, these techniques are usually required in conjunction with domain knowledge to solve picture segmentation problems for a particular domain. In medical imaging applications, image segmentation is crucial because it makes it easier to distinguish between anatomical structures and other areas of interest. The literature offers a number of methods for segmenting medical images. The two fundamental characteristics of intensity values—discontinuity and similarity—are the foundation for most image segmentation methods. The first category uses a method of segmenting an image according to sharp shifts in intensity, such edges. The main techniques in the second group centre around dividing an image into similar parts based on a predetermined set of parameters. Techniques in this category include thresholding, region expanding, and region splitting and merging.

1.12 PSORIASIS IMAGE SEGMENTATION

Image segmentation and classification have become increasingly important in improving patient outcomes and quality of life. A variety of approaches are discussed in this research for the segmentation and classification of psoriasis images, including machine learning algorithms, deep learning techniques, and traditional image processing techniques. Each method has its own advantages and disadvantages. Machine learning algorithms are fast and accurate but require large amounts of data for training. Deep learning techniques can handle complex features but are computationally expensive. Traditional image processing methods are simple but may not be effective in capturing subtle variations in psoriasis lesions. Future directions for research in this field include the development of hybrid approaches that combine the strengths of different methods to achieve better results. In addition, further research is needed to determine whether image segmentation and classification can be used clinically to guide treatment decisions and monitor the progression of the disease. In conclusion, psoriasis image segmentation and classification is a promising area of research that has the potential to significantly improve patient outcomes.

1.13 SEGMENTATION DESIGN FOR MEDICAL IMAGE PROCESSING

The type of segmentation method used and the properties of the medical images determine the problems in designing an efficient segmentation algorithm. Either region-based or edge-based segmentation techniques may be employed. Accurate segmentation in region-based algorithms requires intensity uniformity in the region of interest. For edge-based algorithms to accurately segment data, strong edges are the primary prerequisite. Developing a segmentation algorithm for medical images that exhibits intensity inhomogeneity in region-based models and weak edges in edge-based models is a significant problem.

1.13.1 Feature Extraction

The segmented pre-processed images can be used for feature extraction, which involves performing certain computations over them. Feature extraction is primarily concerned with creating a real-number feature vector that explains the essential characteristics of a medical image supplied. As a result, every single image must also be represented by a point located in feature space, which is a collection of n dimensional spaces. Building a new feature space similar to intrinsic image classifications (malignant/benevolent) that are readily separable in this space is the aim of the feature extraction method. The majority of feature extraction techniques created to extract features from images of skin cancer suggest new characteristics in which a model employs the ABCD rule as applied by doctors in a clinical setting (Patwardhan *et al.* 2013).

Most approaches have been developed in this direction, comparing the features with dermatoscope-collected medical images. Some researchers have incorporated features with specific aims through the feature extraction technique. The decision-making system that analyses the standard images does not often employ these qualities. Numerous research studies have suggested additional aspects for the typical camera photos (Ge *et al.* 2014). These research publications, however, mostly concentrate on either the segmentation and pre-processing tasks or the classification tasks. Finally, the set features are basic which consists of several low-grade features which are combined to approximate the ABCD rule.

1.13.12 Cluster Based Image Segmentation

Among the segmentation algorithms that are now accessible, cluster-based image segmentation is a significant technique. Majority of the existing segmentation algorithms uses the clustering algorithm for performing image segmentation. Generally, clustering algorithms have been applied over the variety of applications with different approaches for handling the different kinds of datasets. The main objective of the clustering algorithms is to place the different clusters from the intensity values that are similar. Moreover, it defined a cluster in the ways such as a cluster is a group of entries that are dislike and the image entities are from the various clusters that are not dis like. Another definition is a cluster is a group of points in the test location like the distance between the two different locations in the cluster that is smaller than the distance between any other two locations in the group and any location not in the cluster. It is also explained the clusters is continuous point of places of a multi-dimensional location which having a relatively high density of regional points that are divided from other such point of regions that are having a relatively less density of regional points.

1.13.3 Classification

Classification (Qiu` et al. 2005) is used to determine whether a test record is part of a particular group of labelled data called training, in order to learn a prediction model named as classifier and to classify it into any one of the classes that have been learned using the learned model referred to as testing. In similar fashion to the training and testing phases of a classification-based medical diagnosis system (Raychaudhuri et al. 2014), classification-based medical diagnosis systems operate in a two-phased manner. Using the provided labelled training data, the training phase in this case learned a classifier. A test record is categorised as "normal" or "disease affected" based on the testing phase. The prediction system based on classification that functions with either single- or multi-class classifiers. Using multi-class classification as a basis for prediction, it may be necessary to include a large number of labelled examples that correspond to the typical classes in the training data (Zollino et al. 2000). A new classifier is used to differentiate between each normal class and the remainder of the classes in such a medical diagnosis method. When no classification algorithm has been able to identify a test image as normal, it has been considered a disease affected image. There are numerous methods in this direction that link the classification algorithm's image prediction to a confidence score. The classification of a test image as disease-affected occurs when no classification algorithm is able to reliably classify the image as normal. It is assumed that all training images have a single class label in single class classification approaches for cancer prediction. The purpose of these methods is to apply a classification technique known as one class classification to learn a discriminative boundary around the normal images. As well, any test image not fitting within the established border is considered to have been altered by cancer.

1.14 PSORIASIS IMAGE CLASSIFICATION

1.14.1 Image Classification

Techniques and their application in psoriasis diagnosis and treatment is still in its early stages, and further research is needed to fully understand its clinical utility. Nevertheless, the ability to accurately segment and classify psoriasis images can provide valuable information for clinicians in guiding treatment decisions and monitoring disease progression. By analyzing the severity of psoriasis lesions and tracking changes over time, clinicians can tailor treatment plans to individual patients and improve overall outcomes. Additionally, the use of image segmentation and classification can reduce subjectivity in diagnosis and improve inter-rater reliability among healthcare providers. Overall, psoriasis image segmentation and classification is a promising field of research for enhancing patient care, even if there is still much to learn about its clinical value.

1.14.2 Methods of Psoriasis Image Classification

Methods of Psoriasis Image Classification have shown promising results in accurately identifying different types and severity levels of psoriasis. This can aid in personalized treatment plans and monitoring disease progression. Additionally, image segmentation techniques can assist in identifying affected areas of the skin, allowing for targeted treatment and assessment of treatment efficacy. It is also possible to improve diagnostic accuracy and reduce human error by utilizing artificial intelligence algorithms and machine learning algorithms in image analysis. However, challenges such as standardization of imaging protocols and large-scale data collection need to be addressed for these methods to be widely implemented in clinical practice. Nonetheless, the potential benefits of image segmentation and classification for psoriasis management make it an exciting area of research with promising future applications.

1.14.3 Advantages and Limitations of Each Method

Advantages and limitations of each method should be carefully considered before choosing the appropriate approach for a specific clinical scenario. Image segmentation allows for precise delineation of psoriatic lesions, enabling accurate measurement of disease severity and tracking of treatment response over time. However, this method can be time-consuming and requires expertise in image analysis. On the other hand, machine learning-based classification algorithms can quickly analyze large datasets and provide automated diagnosis and treatment recommendations. However, these algorithms may lack transparency and interpretability, raising concerns about their reliability and potential biases. Furthermore, the generalizability of these methods to diverse patient populations and imaging modalities needs to be validated before widespread adoption. Despite these challenges, image segmentation and classification hold great promise for improving psoriasis management by providing objective and personalized assessments of disease activity and response to therapy.

1.14.4 Challenges and Solutions in Psoriasis Image Segmentation and Classification

Challenges in psoriasis image segmentation and classification (e.g. variability in psoriasis lesions, overlapping lesions) have led to the development of various solutions. One approach is to use deep learning algorithms that can automatically identify and segment psoriasis lesions from images with high accuracy. Another solution is to incorporate multimodal imaging techniques, such as combining visible light and infrared imaging, to improve lesion detection and classification. Additionally, efforts are being made to standardize imaging protocols and develop robust quality control measures to ensure consistency and reproducibility of results across different imaging platforms. These solutions are crucial for overcoming the challenges in psoriasis image analysis and facilitating the widespread adoption of these techniques in clinical practice. With continued advancements in technology and research, image segmentation and classification have the potential to revolutionize psoriasis management by providing clinicians with objective and personalized assessments of disease activity, leading to more effective treatment strategies for patients.

Solutions to address challenges (e.g. augmentation techniques, multi -stage classification) are being developed to develop the accuracy and efficiency of image segmentation and classification in psoriasis management. These solutions aim to overcome the limitations of traditional methods, such as manual scoring systems, which are subjective and prone to inter-observer variability. By leveraging machine learning algorithms and deep neural networks, researchers are able to extract meaningful features from images and classify them into different categories based on their characteristics. Furthermore, these techniques can be combined with other data sources, such as genetic information or clinical data, to provide a more comprehensive understanding of psoriasis pathogenesis and treatment response. As a result, clinicians can make more informed decisions about patient care and tailor treatment plans to individual needs. While there are still challenges that need to be addressed in implementing these technologies in clinical practice, the potential benefits for patients with psoriasis are significant. With continued research and development, image segmentation and classification could become an essential tool in the management of this chronic skin condition.

1.15 INTRODUCTION OF AUTOMATIC SEGMENTATION AND CLASSIFICATION AS A SOLUTION

There are millions of people worldwide who suffer from psoriasis, which is an autoimmune condition. Accurate diagnosis is crucial for effective treatment, and currently, manual segmentation is the most common method used to distinguish psoriasis lesions from healthy skin tissue. However, this process can be time-consuming and subjective, leading to inconsistencies in diagnosis. Automatic segmentation offers a solution to these limitations by using advanced imaging techniques and algorithms to accurately identify psoriasis lesions. This approach not only improves diagnostic accuracy but also enables more personalized treatment options for patients. By reducing the reliance on manual segmentation, automatic segmentation has the potential to revolutionize psoriasis diagnosis and treatment.

1.15.1 Evaluation of the Automatic Segmentation Model

There is potential for greatly improved patient outcomes if automatic segmentation is used to diagnose and treat psoriasis. By reducing the reliance on manual segmentation, clinicians can save time and increase accuracy in their diagnoses. In previous studies, automatic segmentation techniques have been demonstrated to be effective by using image processing techniques and machine learning algorithms. Data collection and preparation are also important steps in ensuring the accuracy of the model. Results from evaluations of the automatic segmentation model have shown promising results, with high levels of accuracy when compared to manual segmentation. For patients with psoriasis, this has significant implications since accurate diagnosis can dramatically increase the effectiveness of treatment and improve their quality of life. The use of this approach has potential limitations, however, such as issues related to data quality or bias in algorithm development. Future research should focus on addressing these limitations and further improving the accuracy and effectiveness of automatic

1.15.2 Importance of Automatic Classification

Psoriasis is a long-term autoimmune condition affecting the joints, nails, and skin. Red, scaly spots on the skin that can hurt and itch are its defining feature. Although the precise source of psoriasis is uncertain, environmental and genetic factors are thought to play a role. A person's quality of life may be greatly impacted by psoriasis, which can lead to shame, worry, and sadness. Automatic classification of psoriasis can help healthcare professionals diagnose and treat the disease more effectively. By using machine learning algorithms to analyze patient data, doctors can identify patterns in symptoms and develop personalized treatment plans for each individual.

Automatic classification systems have numerous benefits when it comes to diagnosing and treating patients with psoriasis. By analyzing clinical data, these systems can accurately classify patients according to their disease subtype and severity, providing more objective measures of disease activity and response to therapy. This can lead to improved diagnosis and treatment outcomes for patients, as doctors are able to make more informed decisions about their care. Additionally, automatic classification systems can help reduce the workload for healthcare professionals, freeing up time for other important tasks. By analyzing patient data, such as medical history, physical exam findings, and laboratory test results, these systems utilize algorithms to analyze patient information. In order to determine the severity and subtype of a disease, they analyze this data and identify patterns. In general, automatic classification systems may revolutionize the way we diagnose and treat psoriasis, thereby improving patient outcomes and enhancing the efficiency of healthcare delivery.

1.15.3 Applications and Future Directions

Applications of psoriasis image segmentation and classification in clinical practice are vast and varied. One potential use is in the diagnosis of psoriasis, where image analysis could help to distinguish between different types of psoriasis and other skin conditions. The benefit to patients could be improved diagnosis and treatment outcomes as a result of this technology. It is also possible to use image segmentation and classification to monitor the progression of disease over time, which would enable the creation of more tailored treatment plans that would meet the individual needs of each patient. A more objective measure of treatment success could be provided by this technology as well, by applying it to clinical trials for psoriasis. As research in this field continues to advance, it is likely that image segmentation and classification will become an increasingly important tool in the management of psoriasis and other skin conditions.

Potential advancements in psoriasis image segmentation and classification (e.g. using other imaging modalities) may also lead to more personalized treatment plans for patients. Additionally, the integration of machine learning algorithms and artificial intelligence may further enhance the accuracy and efficiency of image analysis in dermatology. This could potentially revolutionize the way skin conditions are diagnosed and treated, ultimately improving patient outcomes. However, it is important to note that these advancements must be balanced with ethical considerations and patient privacy concerns. As such, continued collaboration between medical professionals, researchers, and technology experts will be crucial in ensuring that these tools are used responsibly and ethically in the field of dermatology. Overall, the future of psoriasis image segmentation and classification holds great promise for improving patient care and advancing our understanding of skin conditions.

1.16 MOTIVATION

It is difficult for individuals today to distinguish between types of abnormalities as many skin conditions share the same appearance. In the medical field, numerous applications and technologies have been demonstrated to be useful in medical image analysis, including image processing (Roslan *et al.* 2011), fuzzy logic (Kim & Song 2019), machine learning (Isa *et al.* 2019), artificial neural network (Rawat *et al.* 2018), Convolutional Neural Network (Al-Saffar *et al.* 2017), and optimization algorithm (Zhou *et al.* 2019). Image enhancement, image segmentation, and Image extraction are all handled via image processing. Any procedure used to enhance the appearance of an image is considered an image enhancement. This procedure may also be used to convert an image into a format which is more suitable for machine processing. Recently, Deep Convolutional Neural Networks (CNNs) have gained popularity for feature learning and object categorization. In order to achieve superior performance, it is possible to train a network on large datasets using a GPU with excellent performance. There has been extensive research demonstrating that CNNs are particularly effective at recognizing and categorizing images. However, distinguishing between eczema and psoriasis is difficult because to their comparable appearances.

Most previous approaches have been created with psoriasis skin images acquired against a basic or no backdrop, i.e., limited psoriasis images. A number of issues can exist when imaging with a Smartphone or digital camera, such as motion blur, poor image resolution, noise, etc. A complicated background may also be present in photographs taken by cellphones or digital cameras in outpatient clinics for patients who have psoriasis. Clinical images of psoriasis captured in this manner are frequently unrestricted when used for real-world purposes. There is, however, a possibility that existing image segmentation techniques are not sufficiently strong to handle uncontrolled psoriasis images. Due to this fact, it became necessary to develop an automatic segmentation method as well as an automated classification method for psoriasis skin images to be used in dermatology in order to deal with psoriasis skin images.

1.17 OBJECTIVES

- In order to enhance the performance of the model, an adaptive chimp optimization algorithm based on a CNN is used to automatically segment psoriasis skin images.

- To diagnose psoriasis skin disease by segmenting images of infected skin.

- To classify an image as normal or psoriasis using double-pathway cascaded convolution neural network, that enhance the classification performance.

- To Making it simple for people to identify skin irregularities early would help to prevent serious infections in patients.

1.18 ORGANIZATION OF THE THESIS

Chapter 2 explains the recent literature review related to psoriasis diagonasis and various image segmentation and classification techniques

Chapter 3 explains the problem statement and contribution of this research work.

Chapter 4 presents an Adaptive Chimp Optimization Algorithm (AChOA) based convolutional neural network (CNN) for automatic segmentation of psoriasis skin images. After preprocessing, the AChOA-CNN model is used to segment input images. As the CNN weights and biases are optimized by AChOA, the output images are segmented.

Chapter 5 presents efficient automatic psoriasis disease classification using double-pathway cascaded convolution neural network DPCCNN with single-pathway CNN, which extracts both local and global features simultaneously to classify an image as normal or psoriasis. As a part of this study, cascaded CNNs are used, where the output of one CNN is used as a further input to subsequent CNNs. Adaptive crocodile optimization (ACO) is used to optimize the weight values in the FCL to enhance classification performance.

Chapter 6 summarizes the work provided in this thesis and identifies opportunities for future research.

CHAPTER 2

LITERATURE SURVEY

2.1 OUTLINE

The automatic segmentation and categorization of skin images with psoriasis is thoroughly examined in this chapter. Examining current approaches for image segmentation and classification in psoriasis diagnosis, along with any possible advantages and disadvantages, is the goal of this review of the research. Understanding these techniques can help to increase the precision and efficacy of psoriasis diagnosis and therapy, which will eventually enhance the quality of life for people who have the condition.

2.2 SURVEY ON AUTOMATIC SEGMENTATION OF PSORIASIS SKIN IMAGES

Narendra Londhe *et al.* (2020) suggested a completely automated CADx system for psoriasis based on deep learning. All three processes were smoothly incorporated into a single framework in the presented CADx system, and the entire intervention was executed automatically with no manual involvement. There were two advantages to using U-Net for autonomous segmentation. In this way, the system was improved in terms of automation and dependability. In addition, the severity assessment was improved as well. Compared to current state-of-the-art methods, this modified VGG model performed better for binary and multiclass classification, resulting in a higher classification accuracy and smaller training set. An expanded dataset was utilised to test this methodology. The method was used on a bigger dataset, and by adjusting the data size, its dependability was also confirmed.

An algorithm based on deep convolutional neural networks was developed by Guo-Shiang Lin *et al.* (2021) for diagnosing uncontrolled psoriasis images. In order to handle images of psoriasis, the authors used a network of features pyramids, protonets, and prediction heads - You Only Look At CoefficienTs (YOLACT). Multiscale feature maps were created by using the FPN, while backbone maps were extracted from images using the backbone network. With the help of the prediction head, the authors were able to predict the categorization information for objects, the bounding box information, as well as the mask coefficients. Protonet prototypes were used in conjunction with mask coefficients to forecast an object's pixel-level form. Transfer learning was used to retrain YOLACT++ using a pretrained model in order to do instance segmentation for uncontrolled psoriasis images.

A fully automated method for identifying psoriasis lesions from digital images captured in an uncontrolled setting with a non-uniform backdrop has been developed by Narendra Londhe et al. (2021). This method uses deep learning techniques based on transfer learning to identify psoriasis lesions from digital images. This scheme can automatically separate psoriasis lesions without the need for preprocessing or human feature engineering. An analysis of the segmentation performance using the indicated method was conducted using five-fold cross-validation. The recommended method demonstrated effective and promising segmentation performance with an average DI of 0.948 and a JI of 0.901. Additionally, the authors tested the model with various picture sizes, batch sizes, and transfer learning factors. The approach indicated unsuitable for automated and objective assessment of psoriasis lesions in order to calculate psoriasis area.

George *et al.* (2020) offered a detailed assessment of skin segmentation methods for psoriasis images. For 2D psoriasis images, the authors developed pixel-based skin segmentation methods. A significant concern noted by the authors of this study was the overlap between pixels from psoriasis and pixels from nonskin. This increases the difficulty of the segmentation process. This study presented four high-performing techniques: (i) an explicit thresholding method based on the CbCr decision boundary; (ii) Bayesian classification followed by a decision tree; (iii) Bayesian classification with majority voting; and (iv) Bayesian classification with binary OR. They also presented a detailed examination of the various colour bands and how they affected the skin segmentation process. Furthermore, the segmentation results were enhanced through post-processing based on morphological factors. The system shown incapable of dealing with complicated backgrounds.

An ML-based psoriasis skin segmentation method was developed by Yasmeen George *et al.* (2017), followed by morphological operations for refining this method. To accomplish this, the authors employed seven machine learning (ML) classifiers, including SVM, K-NN, NB, DT, RF, Adaboost, and MLP. The experimental findings provided in this work reveal that virtually all individual classifiers accurately recognised redness and "Tatto" related pixels, however most classifiers fail to distinguish white scales as skin regions. These issues were addressed in two steps by the authors: 1) the skin maps acquired from the seven separate classifiers are aggregated by a committee of classifiers based on majority voting, and 2) morphological operations are employed to refine the resulting skin map. The experimental data indicates that their gain was substantial. A commonly used dataset for facial skin was used to train and test all classifiers in order to examine the robustness of the idea put forth.

Datchakorn Tancharoen (2019) and colleagues presented an automated technique for segmenting regions of interest that can objectively determine the PASI area score. K-mean clustering was used in this work to separate the region of interest (ROI) from the normal skin and remove background from the skin region. The colour space analysis was carried out using YCbCr and YIQ. Ten skin imaging samples from the hospital's experimental database were examined for this study. The recommended algorithm performed well in segmenting the psoriasis area and measuring the region of interest with realistic precision for diagnosing psoriasis, based on the results.

Yasmeen George *et al.* (2019) presented a novel, robust, reliable, and fully automated method for measuring lesions in two-dimensional skin scans. It was suggested that a scale severity evaluation method may be applied to two-dimensional psoriasis skin scans by the authors of the study. By exploiting superpixels as key points, they extract lesion features based on the bag-of-visual-words (BoVWs) paradigm. The BoVWs model was developed by employing a clustering technique with specific local characteristics drawn from a collection of key-points to construct a vocabulary with a given word count (i.e. codebook size). An ML classifier with three classes was then constructed using support vector machines (SVMs) and random forests (RFs). In addition, they examine eight different descriptors of texture and color at the local level. The offered technique does not require the use of a ground truth for the scale. Unfortunately, the lack of annotated images made the system unworkable, forcing them to restrict the scale score to three rather than five groups.

By combining segmentation and risk categorization, Vimal K Shrivastava *et al.* (2017) established a fully automated system for evaluating the severity of psoriasis disease in a multi-class setting. Researchers used a

Bayesian approach to segment psoriatic lesions autonomously and have created nine risk stratification systems with three classifiers and three feature selection methods each. All nine of these pRAS systems had been thoroughly inspected.A99.84% classification accuracy was achieved using the combination of FDR feature selection and the SVM classifier. Three performance indices were used to evaluate each of the nine pRAS systems: aggregate feature effect, feature retention power, and reliability index. All systems worked flawlessly together, achieving high levels of stability and dependability.

PsLSNet, based on a modified U-Net architecture, was presented by Narendra D Londhe *et al.* (2019). Automatic spatial data extraction is performed using a 29-layer deep fully convolutional network. The U-Net architecture consisted of two paths that are coupled in a U-shape: contracting and extracting. The convolutional neural network that was built was able to segment lesions even in challenging situations, like poor acquisition conditions and the presence of artefacts. It also offered quicker training by lowering covariate shift by batch normalisation implementation. The degree of psoriasis could not be determined by the method, though.

In order to express hue and chroma information, Anabik Pal *et al.* (2017) suggested a bi-variate circular-linear distribution mixture. In the framework, different margins were handled for different mixture components, and a circular copula was used to merge the distribution of two linear and circular variables. To segregate psoriatic plaques in skin images, the authors used hue and chroma information. There was a heterogeneous distribution of chroma in a picture of skin. Additionally, the combined distribution of hue and chroma displayed multi-modal characteristics. To achieve automated plaque localization, they use a statistical model based on the colour information of the segmented areas after segmentation. As demonstrated by the experimental results, this segmentation model performs better than numerous competing supervised and unsupervised approaches in recognizing psoriatic plaque locations in skin images. Despite its effectiveness, the approach does not provide a model for predicting the distribution of skin colors according to colour tone and geographic region.

The major focus of this research is the measurement of psoriasis severity. Yasmeen George *et al.* (2017) presented a completely automated system for segmenting psoriasis lesions with scales and erythema. The image collection utilised in this study was the biggest used in psoriasis segmentation to date. Based on the findings of this study, this method was found to segment psoriasis images reliably and effectively, regardless of the resolution of the image, the lesion shape, size, or severity, or the presence of hairs on the skin. To segregate psoriasis, the authors employed unsupervised approaches (superpixel and K-means algorithms). To enhance the segmentation of individual single superpixel scales, multiscale and image fusion approaches were used. Smoothing or other preprocessing procedures were excluded in this method.

To detect skin disorders more accurately, Arora et al. (2012) aimed to reduce the time needed. Therefore, they were able to produce automatic dermoscopic image segmentation using a deep learning system. Modeling was conducted using a modified U-net architecture. As part of the U-net, Group Normalisation was applied to the encoder and decoder levels. In the skip link, Gates noticed small features that were later validated by Tversky. A loss function was used as a measure of yield loss. Group normalisation was used to obtain feature maps in the study. An improvement in recall and accuracy was achieved by using the Tversky Loss, based on the Tversky index. By implementing these tactics, the researchers improved accuracy and Jaccard.

Anabik Pal *et al.* (2018) proposed a method for automatically and reliably segmenting epidermal and dermal layers in psoriasis skin biopsy images as a first step in analyzing images of psoriasis histopathology. It was demonstrated that the authors' research can be viewed as a study to develop an efficient machine-aided tool for the interpretation of psoriasis biopsy images by integrating several image processing and computer vision techniques. In comparison to conventional feature-based classifiers such as the K-Nearest Neighbor (KNN), the Support Vector Machine (SVM), and the Random Forest (RF), the performance of these architectures has been compared to that of the conventional hand-crafted classifiers. Simple Linear Iterative Clustering (SLIC) generates super-pixels that are categorised using deep models. According to the experimental findings, when compared to the conventional techniques, deep neural networks might provided effective segmentation algorithms.

A method of automating manual segmentation of images was proposed by Khatibi *et al.* (2021). They have therefore achieved automatic segmentation of images for vitiligo spot diagnosis. In raw images, the authors detected vitiligo patches using a stack ensemble of deep learning and conventional segmentation methods. In contrast to manual segmentation, unsupervised segmentation does not require prior knowledge. As a result of the recommended technique, they enhanced their accuracy, sensitivity, and specificity.

In order to improve the accuracy of psoriasis skin image segmentation, Karthick Panneerselvam *et al.* (2023) employed a convolutional neural network approach. Psoriasis input images were adjusted and scaled during a preprocessing phase. A final application of the IGEO technique used the preprocessed images as input into an optimized CNN, and the bias and weight parameters were improved using the IGEO technique.

The GEO algorithm's search capabilities were also enhanced by a confusing sequence created by a tent map. The threshold module was used to remove artefacts from segmented images. Based on the results of the study, this IGEO-CNN-based segmentation model obtained 98% accuracy, 92% JI, and 97% DC. However, the system does not take diseases detection models into consideration.

Birkenfeld *et al.* (2020) developed the computer-aided classifier method to detect worrisome pigmented lesions. A machine learning classification system was developed by the authors to distinguish suspicious pigmented lesions (SPLs) from non-suspicious pigmented lesions (non-SPLs). As part of their investigation, the scientists examined 133 individuals suffering from a variety of skin lesions. According to the imaging, all lesions are evaluated by a dermatologist who is board-certified. It has been determined that the sensitivity for suspicious pigmented lesions is 100% based on the testing set. In the context of population-based screening, this computer-aided classifier method proved to be extremely beneficial.

The segmentation of medical images is one of the most important aspects of image analysis. A deep learning system for segmenting medical images, CE-Net, has been presented by Zaiwang Gu *et al.* (2019). The CE-Net feature encoder is different from the U-Net encoder, as it is based on a pretrained ResNet block. ResNet modified UNet framework was merged with a newly dense atrous convolution block and residual multi-kernel pooling so as to capture more high-level features and retain more spatial information. Our model can be fine-tuned using additional training data and manual ground truth to apply it to a new application after fine-tuning it with additional training data. The results of their experiments demonstrated that the suggested technique could improve the segmentation of medical images in a wide variety of tasks, such as optic disc segmentation, retinal vascular detection, pulmonary segmentation, cell contour segmentation, and retinal OCT layer segmentation. This approach, however, has not been tested on 3D images.

Narendra D Londhe *et al.* (2020) stated a unique psoriasis image segmentation approach for lesion diagnosis based on automated clustering. The authors combined traditional clustering algorithms (K-means and FCM) with well-known swarm intelligence-based methods (SO, ABC, ACO, and PSO). They constructed and evaluated their suggested approach using a collection of 780 psoriasis images from 74 individual patients. The results reveal that the novel segmentation algorithms outperform traditional clustering strategies significantly. Furthermore, it was discovered that SO outperformed ACO, PSO, and ABC in terms of lesion identification accuracy.

2.3 SURVEY ON AUTOMATIC PSORIASIS DISEASE CLASSIFICATION

A single deep learning strategy was used in previous methodologies, which did not classify diverse forms of psoriasis; instead, Saad Jawaid Khan *et al.* (2022) devised a deep learning methodology for this purpose. According to the BFL NTU dataset, 172 images depict normal skin, while the Dermnet collection contains 301 photographs depicting psoriasis. In order to extract colour, texture, and form features, input images were preprocessed, including data enhancement, enhancement, and segmentation. A combination of Long Short-Term Memory (LSTM) and Convolutional Neural Network (CNN) were used as deep learning techniques. The classification models were trained using 80 percent of the images. It should be noted that earlier state-of-the-art efforts used different datasets than those used in this study, and they achieved greater accuracy. The study did not assess the severity and area of psoriasis (PASI).

Saptarshi Chatterjee *et al.* (2019) suggested an integrated computer-aided technique for detecting skin disorders. The form, color, texture, and uneven border of the skin lesion were analyzed in order to determine a number of quantitative parameters prior to categorization. In order to quantify the texture information, fractal-based regional texture analysis (FRTA) and graylevel co-occurrence matrices (GLCM) were applied. Support vector machines and radial basis functions were used to evaluate the classification performance. A 99.65% classification accuracy is obtained for BCC, 97.54% for dysplastic nevi, and 98.99% for melanoma, respectively, in the experimental analysis, however, the feature dimensionality space was larger for BCC.

The Deep Convolutional Neural Network (DCNN) classifier was proposed by Dong-Hyun Kim *et al.*(2020) for the diagnosis of skin disorders. Inception-ResNet-v2, ResNet-50, and Inception-V3 networks are included in the convolutional neural Med Biol Eng Comput network classifier. A full resolution convolutional network (FrCN) was used to segment the borders of skin lesions from the entire dermoscopy image set. To evaluate the performance of convolutional neural network classifiers in the categorization of skin diseases, the ISIC 2016, ISIC 2017, and ISIC 2018 datasets were used. However, the labelled skin lesion images used for deep learning network training and testing were still limited in size.

Saeid Afshare *et al.* (2021) reported a hybrid approach for diagnosing psoriasis that included GA and SVM. The technique also chose gene signatures. The model was evaluated against a publicly available gene expression dataset. A hybrid model was used to select 181 probe sets from the initial 54,675 probes, which resulted in a prediction accuracy of 100% over the test set. Ten hub genes were identified based on the protein-protein interaction network. There were nine significant modules containing the ten genes identified. Results indicated that the genetic algorithm significantly improved the performance of the SVM classifier, indicating that the proposed model has the capability of identifying relevant gene expression profiles as the best features for classifying data.

According to Chatterjee *et al.* (2019), multi-label classification algorithms can be used to detect skin pathologies such as SK, BCC, nevus, psoriasis, and melanoma. Feature extraction was performed using cross-spectrum and cross-correlation techniques. Using kernel patches and visual consequences, spectral and spatial feature extraction was taught. Skin lesions were classified using a multi-label ensemble multiclass classification method, including epidermal, benign melanocytic, and benign melanocytic. The classification performance indices demonstrate that utilizing the disclosed feature extraction approach, all of the sickness classes under consideration can be identified with a high degree of sensitivity and accuracy at each phase.

Qin *et al.* (2020) developed a system for medical image analysis that utilizes GAN technology to classify skin lesions. As a result of the GAN-based data augmentation strategy, the performance of skin lesion categorization was improved. A high-quality image of the skin lesion can be obtained by adjusting the discriminator and generator. Several quantitative parameters are used to evaluate the performance of skin lesion style-based GANs, including recall, precision, inception distance (FID), and inception score (IS). According to the experimental analysis, the average precision was 96.6%, the specificity was 74.3%, the sensitivity was 83.2%, and the accuracy was 95.2%. However, the system lacked a better feature extraction strategy and had poor classifier performance.

An evaluation of the categorization of Psoriasis skin condition using a Convolutional Neural Network was proposed by Rosniza Roslan *et al.* (2020). The Psoriasis Image Library, the International Psoriasis Council

(IPC), and DermNet NZ provided a total of 187 images of plaque psoriasis and guttate psoriasis. Psoriasis skin disease categorization was performed using a Convolutional Neural Network (CNN). In this study, CNN was demonstrated to be capable of accurately predicting Plaque and Guttate Psoriasis skin diseases, respectively, with accuracy rates of 82.9% and 72.4%. In addition to being beneficial for medical dermatology, this study was also useful for medical dermatology practices, particularly those dealing with Psoriasis.

Bajwa *et al.* (2020) presented a deep neural network (DNN) for identifying skin diseases. DermNet and ISIC Archive databases were used to choose skin disease images. On DermNet, the authors also established a new state-of-the-art result for 23-ary categorization. Most medical image databases absence generally include non-visual information. Even so, if such extra information is included, DNNs are capable of using it and increasing classification performance, as demonstrated by this experiment with leveraging disease taxonomy to considerably enhance classification accuracy. The experimental findings show improved repeatability and accuracy. However, it required more time to execute.

A proper classification of psoriasis lesions is essential in order to provide an early and accurate diagnosis, and normal and psoriasis cells exhibit distinct gene expression patterns. A machine learning model was developed using gene expression data collected from microarrays and 35 expression characteristics associated with psoriasis by Nguyen Quoc Khanh Le *et al.* (2021). The performance of the model based on the 35 previously stated characteristics exceeded the performance of existing state-of-the-art classifiers in 5fold cross-validation tests, with an average accuracy of 98.3%, recall of 98.6%, and precision of 98%. Two sets of psoriasis patients were also used to validate the model, and the results showed significant improvements in performance. These findings indicated that their 35 expression profiles were found as important factors for categorising samples as lesion or nonlesion.

An automatic erythema severity grading method based on semi-supervised computer-aided analysis was presented by Yasmeen George *et al.* (2018). First, a brand-new image representation technique was incorporated in the unsupervised stage. Based on the dictionary developed by the authors, local features were extracted from the sparse representation. In order to obtain the final image representation vector, we used an aggregation approach on the local characteristics. During the supervised phase, several multi-class machine learning (ML) classifiers were developed to grade the severity of erythema. Following the discussion of the suggested system, a comparison was made between it and two well-known unsupervised feature extraction algorithms, such as the bag of visual words model (BoVWs) and the pretrained AlexNet algorithm. In this study, a set of 676 images depicting psoriasis has been used.

An entire-stage data augmentation strategy for DCNN has been proposed by Zheng *et al.* (2020), improving its accuracy in natural image categorization. It is the purpose of data augmentation to ensure that the network can extract structural information from samples during the training process and eventually converge to a optimal position. The purpose of data augmentation in testing is to reduce dependency on a single network by acting as a model ensemble. In the training and testing phases, data augmentation can improve network generalization and optimize performance. According to the model, it achieves accuracy of 93.41% and 70.22% when applied to coarse-grained datasets (CIFAR10) and fine-grained datasets (CIFAR100). The system requires more training time and higher reasoning costs.

A unique loss function was developed by Anabik Pal *et al.* (2018) with the goal of making CNN appropriate for ordinal categorization and utilised for automated psoriatic plaque severity evaluation. The use of a loss function was a challenging undertaking. The severity of the plaque was assessed by training separate CNNs for erythema (redness), scaling (silverness), and induration (elevation). In order to evaluate performance, mean accuracy (MA), mean absolute error (MAE), and Kendall's beta were used. According on the experimental findings, the suggested ordinal classification strategy works better than the established methods.

An algorithm for automating modulation categorization based on two levels of data augmentation was presented by Qinghe Zheng *et al.* (2021). The authors demonstrated how data augmentation was computed using a model ensemble during the testing phase. The STFT and IFFT are used to aid signal expansion and add variations while keeping critical features in order to resemble the global input space as closely as feasible. In addition, they showed that the augmentation of data during the test step might be interpreted as an implicit ensemble of models. The majority voting approach improved stability and classification performance. With data augmentation used during training and testing, the suggested technique achieves a classification accuracy of 58.75%.

Arunkumar *et al.* (2022) developed the MobileNet machine learning architecture, which was built on depthwise separable convolutions, to detect the kind of psoriasis condition. With the aid of the Keras Image Data Generator function, the input images were divided into 224 pixels by 224 pixels in the preprocessing stage. In the following phase, these segmented images were provided as input to 28 layers of the rebuilt MobileNet architecture. The input images were subjected to a number of convolutions and depth-wise separable convolutions layers. The network's nonlinearity was added using the rectified linear activation function. The network was trained using the Adam optimizer algorithm. The categorical cross-entropy was used to assess the accuracy of the experimental findings in relation to previous work on the categorization of psoriatic conditions.

An innovative pCAD method for the automatic categorization of the skin disease psoriasis was presented by Narendra Londhe *et al.* (2015) and demonstrated the potency of colour characteristics by utilising 14 different colour spaces. This system was expanded to include grayscale features on its own or shown how it might alter its categorization methods when colour and grayscale information were combined. The use of a PCA-based feature selection criterion without changing the real or original feature values improved the model's simplicity. In order to ensure sensitivity, specificity, correctness, and dependability while utilised in all three setups—color space, grayscale space, and combined colour and grayscale spaces—the total system, known as pCAD, passed all important data mining procedures. The hypothesis was established and supported by an analysis of the effectiveness of the colour characteristic.

Skin lesions can result from a variety of different disorders, but some of them require prompt attention and subsequent treatment. A skin image processing will be requested by the doctor in order to diagnose a skin lesion. To assist this activity, Balaji *et al.* (2020) introduced a unique skin image segmentation technique in this study, which was then classified using a naive Bayes classifier. The segmentation method for graphs that was put out in this study had the advantages of being practical efficient, labelling that was globally optimum, incorporating various cues and restrictions, being numerically resilient, and allowing for unlimited topological features of areas. The approach suggested here dynamically modified the seeds across iterations to produce superior segmentation results than many other comparable methods, but the old methods had the limitation that the seed pixels could not alter their labels afterwards.

Based on clinical images and patient data, Simegn *et al.* (2022) employed DL to determine the skin conditions that the patients suffered. An automated method was created that leverages a deep learning pre-trained mobilenet-v2 model to diagnose five common skin conditions based on clinical photographs and patient data. Various smartphone cameras were used to take clinical images while the patient was being registered. A variety of data pre-processing and augmentation techniques were used to enhance the model's performance before training. Using this method, the common five skin diseases were classified with 97.5% accuracy, 97.7% sensitivity, and 97.7% precision.

2.4 SUMMARY

The literature survey conducted in this study highlights the key findings from selected studies on psoriasis image segmentation and classification. The comparison of different techniques used for image segmentation and classification reveals that there is no one-size-fits-all approach to this process. Each technique has its own strengths and weaknesses, which must be considered when selecting the most appropriate method for a particular application. The discussion of limitations and future research directions emphasizes the need for further investigation into the development of more accurate and efficient methods for psoriasis image segmentation and classification.

CHAPTER 3

PROBLEM STATEMENT AND CONTRIBUTION

3.1 PROBLEM STATEMENT

Psoriasis is a persistent, genetic disease. It is virtually always a game changer, limiting people's activities, sending them into desperation, and raising their risk for illnesses. Early psoriasis detection is essential since it can help avoid problems like joint damage and heart disease. As a result, improving outcomes for persons with psoriasis requires increasing awareness of the significance of early identification and treatment. The sole way to diagnose a disease manually is to looks at the skin's surface, however this method has several drawbacks due to the unreliable, repeatable, and unquantifiable nature of human eyesight. There is an abundance of information contained in the medical imaging data that may be obtained utilising different skin disease image analysis techniques. An accurate diagnosis of the condition is necessary for planning the diagnostic. Due to recent advancements in the field of medical imaging, several algorithms and artificial intelligence models may now be able to address imaging problems more successfully.

For decades, a number of machine learning-based techniques for autonomous skin disease image interpretation have been presented. The existing methods extract hand-crafted image attributes, such as edge, form, texture, and colour, depending on the understanding of the target domain. This knowledge-driven approach has drawbacks, such as the likelihood that non-experts lack the medical knowledge necessary to build an effective feature extraction approach and the fact that handmade features often perform poorly in complex circumstances.

Due to the complexity of the image capture technology, segmenting skin disease images remains a difficult challenge. An efficient approach for denoising and deblurring is required for various skin diseases, as the majority of images are damaged by noises and abnormalities induced by the different acquisition techniques. It is a tremendous task to get a classifier to classify skin diseases more accurately when the conditions are bad.

A variety of techniques have been used to segment the areas of psoriasis in the images, including SVMs, random forests, etc. It is imperative to segment the region using features before training the machine learning framework. The problem with these feature extraction techniques is that they do not preserve the spatial resolution of an image, which increases the likelihood of incorrect recognition when difficult conditions are present.

Challenges of image segmentation

- Utilization of unique segmentation algorithm for all sort of psoriasis skin images.
- The selection of appropriate quantitative measurement metrics for evaluating segmentation methods for various types of input images is essential.
- Determining the optimal objective function or correct predefined criterion.
- Solving the objective function of such methods can be done only by non-deterministic models which are very difficult.

- Segmentation of color input medical image is very difficult task than gray level image.
- Using segmentation algorithms on colour images and assessing how well they work are regarded as challenging tasks in image processing.

For detection, localization, and tracking, skin detection is a reliable and practical event. A trade-off between response time and proper classification rate is a crucial requirement for autonomous skin detection systems. Typically, skin colour is used as a characteristic for skin detection. Different color space, cluster methods are studied and applied with various parameters to segment the skin pixels. With the advent of automated systems, however, skin psoriasis can be identified by lesion regions having a clear boundary and color variation. The following issues are dealt in the earliest method of detections.

(i) There is a risk that small-sized lesions could likely be misclassified as moles or scars.

(ii) The complexion of the skin is another issue. In dark-skinned people, the color of the lesion closely resembles their normal skin color.

(iii) In the early stages, since the surface smoothness of the skin is not affected, surface variations between normal skin and the affected portion are minimal.

3.2 CONTRIBUTION OF THE THESIS

Phase 1:

Recently, deep learning techniques like CNN have been able to partition psoriasis images by extracting characteristics from the input image.

The segmentation approach based on CNN performs better, although accuracy might yet be improved.

- An optimized CNN is presented here for segmenting images of psoriasis. An optimization of the weights and biases of the convolutional layer improves the performance of the CNN. These weight and bias parameters were determined using the Adaptive Chimp Optimization Algorithm (AChOA).

- An improved search performance can be achieved by including a chaotic sequence-based tent map in the ChOA algorithm. Using the threshold module, the defects in the segmented image are then removed.

- Several measures of accuracy, precision, recall, and F-measure are reported for the proposed strategy (AChOA+CNN) in comparison to CNN, SVM, ANN, and RF.

Phase 2:

To avoid the problem, in this research automatic psoriasis disease classification using a double- pathway cascaded convolution neural network is proposed.

- The three steps of the suggested methodology are pre-processing, data augmentation, and classification.

- The noises are first pre-processed to improve the input image. Preprocessing is followed by data augmentation.

- The DPCCNN classifier is then used to determine if an image is normal or has psoriasis. This paradigm considers a CNN's output as extra input information for future CNNs.

- The weight values provided in the DPCCNN classifier are ideally chosen utilizing an adaptive crocodile optimization method to improve the performance of the classifier. This conventional crocodile optimization method has been improved with levy flying behaviour. Precision, recall, and F-score are used to assess the success of the proposed approach.

CHAPTER 4

AUTOMATIC SEGMENTATION OF PSORIASIS SKIN IMAGES USING ADAPTIVE CHIMP OPTIMIZATION ALGORITHM BASED CNN

4.1 INTRODUCTION

This has an Skin diseases such as psoriasis can affect specific areas or the entire body, regardless of one's age or gender. The majority of cases of psoriasis are genetic, because the skin grows faster and for longer periods of time than normal skin, according to Tancharoen *et al.* (2019), Lu Juan *et al.* (2012), George *et al.* (2016) impact on the patients lives as well; they feel completely embarrassed and ashamed as a result of the constant tingling and horrible physical appearance. As a consequence of computer vision's ability to segment images of affected skin in recent years, it has become an important tool in the detection of psoriatic skin diseases. Psoriasis-affected skin has been segmented by machine learning methods published by several researchers. In spite of this, it is necessary to improve accuracy and time consumption. The objective of this research is to automatically generate segmentation methods for psoriatic skin images using a convolutional neural network (CNN) based on the Adaptive Chimp Optimization Algorithm. Using the AChOA-CNN model after preprocessing the input images, the CNN's weight and bias values are optimized by the AChOA. Through altering the chaotic sequence according to the tent map, the ChOA algorithm's search capability is enhanced. Finally, the threshold module removes distortions from the segmented output images. Simulation allows us to achieve 97% accuracy.

4.2 METHODOLOGY

Existing Methods for Automatic Segmentation of Psoriasis Skin Images.

4.3 SUPPORT VECTOR MACHINE (SVM)

A relatively new categorization method created by Vapnik and his group at AT&T Bell Laboratories is the support vector machine (SVM). By balancing the accuracy of the training data with the machine's capacity, SVM strives to achieve the best generalisation performance. A number of factors contribute to its development, including the bias-variance tradeoff as well as overfitting. A variety of applications have been developed using it, including identifying handwritten digits, recognizing objects, detecting faces in photographs, and categorizing text. In most circumstances, the performance of SVM has been shown to be comparable or superior to that of competing approaches (Burges 1998). As a primary principle of SVM, the classes are separated using a hyperplane surface in order to maximize the margin between them. Using SVM as an application of the Structural Risk Minimization principle (Vapnik 1982), a decision function is reduced in generalisation error by the reduction of structural risk minimization. The classification of SVM is based on Vapnik (1995), Osuna et al. (2000), and Burges (1998), which identify three types: linearly separable, nonseparable, and nonlinearly separable.

Because Support Vector Machines (SVM) enables accurate classification from small training sets, they are gaining popularity as an alternative to standard image classification techniques. Automation of parameter tweaking, however, is not a universal solution for SVM issues. Support vector machines (SVMs) have attracted a great deal of attention and importance and are actively applied to various domains (Himani Bhavsar & Mahesh Panchal 2012). The foundations of SVMs are structural risk minimization and statistical learning theory. Their goal is to locate the decision borders, sometimes called hyperplanes, at the point where the best possible class separation is achieved. Greater separation between the instances on each side and the dividing hyperplane is produced by maximising the margin. SVM is robust to handle data dimensionality (Liu *et al.* 2010). Training time for different SVMs is not constant, hence researchers are constantly striving to develop an efficient training method, resulting in a variety of differently designed algorithms, most of which are acceptable for linear spaces. Through kernel function projections and linear classification in the feature space, SVM can be extended to learn non-linear decision functions. Most computers are unable to store the generated feature space since it is significantly larger than the dataset in question. SVMs were designed for binary classification. It is possible that SVM can be enhanced to handle multi-class situations. Decomposing a multi-class classification into a two-class type makes it acceptable for SVM-based analysis.

4.3.1 SVM for Classification

In classifying data, SVMs are useful approaches. However, they can sometimes produce undesirable results, since they are more difficult to implement than neural networks. Training and testing data are often included in classification tasks. Each instance has a single target value and multiple attributes (Duda & Hart 1973). As a result of the attributes of the data instances in the testing set, the SVM creates a model which enables it to predict the target value of the data (Chen *et al.* 2017). SVM classification is one example of a supervised learning application. Known labels aid in determining whether or not the system is functioning properly. This data can be used to train the system to perform appropriately or to signal the expected answer, thereby confirming the system's accuracy. Detection of entities that have a close relationship to the recognised classes is a step in the SVM classification process. We refer to this as feature extraction or feature selection. Even in situations when it is not required to predict unknown data, feature selection and SVM classification can be useful in conjunction. The key sets they identify can be used to identify the processes and sets that contribute to the differentiation of classes, according to Chen et al. (2017).

4.3.2 SVM for Regression

Chen *et al.* (2017), they explain how the loss function needs to be altered to incorporate a distance measure in order to identify key sets involved in the processes that separate classes. A linear regression can be used as well as a nonlinear regression. In linear models, the loss functions are primarily quadratic, Huber, and e-intensive. A non-linear model is usually needed for data modelling, just as for classification problems. To perform linear regression, a non-linear mapping can be used, similar to the non-linear SVC method. To address the issue of the dimensionality curse, the kernel technique is employed once again. As part of the regression approach, prior knowledge of the problem and the distribution of noise is taken into account. Several studies have demonstrated that Huber's robust loss function is a suitable substitute when such information is not available (Cortes & Vapnik 1995).

4.3.3 Applications of SVM

SVM has been found to be effective in solving pattern categorization problems. To apply the Support Vector technique to a particular practical scenario, it is necessary to solve certain questions related to the problem formulation and design. Selecting the right kernel for a given application is one of the biggest issues (Burges 1998). Default settings include common choices like a polynomial or Gaussian kernel; however, more complex kernels will be required if these options are not successful or if the inputs consist of discrete structures. Kernels provide a computer with the descriptive language needed to analyze data by automatically establishing a feature space. The fundamental components of the system are assembled once the kernel and optimisation criterion have been chosen. Here are a few examples to illustrate the point. Classifying texts is a process of categorizing them according to their content. Documents can be assigned to more than one category, so this is not a multiclass classification problem. There are several binary classification tasks involved in this process, one for each category. The Mercer kernel can be built using a standard representation of text for information retrieval purposes, as suggested by Osuna et al. (1997). It is true that the kernels in some way include a similarity metric between instances, and one might assume that experts in a particular application domain have already established appropriate similarity metrics, particularly in fields such as generative models and information retrieval (Veropoulos *et al.* 1999).

Although extremely high dimensional representations offer difficulties for Support Vector Machines, the excessive dimensionality of the input causes classical classification algorithms to perform badly when applied directly. Similar to the word categorization methods discussed below, picture classification can be tackled in a similar manner, and in both cases, linear hard margin machines are frequently capable of strong generalisation. An application of support vector machines to handwritten character recognition was the first to be tested in real-world conditions. In addition to testing SVMs in single classes, these data have also been used to test SVMs in multi-classes. SVMs are interesting for comparison with other classifiers, however, it is also interesting to compare several SVMs with one another [82]. Regardless of the kernel chosen, they exhibit almost the same performance and many of their support vectors are shared. Even without any comprehensive prior knowledge, SVM is capable of outperforming these systems (Osuna *et al.* 1997).

4.3.4 Strength and Weakness of SVM

The simplicity of training is one of SVM's key benefits. Local ideals don't exist, in contrast to neural networks. It can effectively handle the trade-off between classifier error and complexity, and it scales to high dimensional data with reasonable ease. The requirement for a strong kernel function is one of the flaws.

In the development of classifiers, SVM is an effective method. By using one or more feature vectors (6), it is possible to predict labels between two classes. Decision boundaries, or hyperplanes, are positioned so that they are as far away as possible from the closest data points in each class. A support vector is a set of points that are closest together. The following steps can be taken to use a labelled training dataset: $(x_1, y_1), \ldots, (x_n, y_n), x_i \in R^d$ and

$$y_i \in (-1, +1) \tag{4.1}$$

It is assumed that x_i represents a feature vector, while y_i represents the class label (positive or negative) associated with a training compound *i*. Thus, a hyper plane that is optimal can be defined as follows:

$$wx^T + b = 0 \tag{4.2}$$

The above equation uses w to represent the weight vector, x to represent the feature vector input, and b to represent the bias vector. The following inequalities would be satisfied by w and b based on all elements of the training set:

$$wx_i^T + b \geq +1 \tag{4.3}$$

if $y_i = 1$

$$wx_i^T + b \leq -1 \text{ if } y_i = -1 \tag{4.4}$$

To maximise the margin $1/\|w\|^2$ and divide the data with a hyperplane, a SVM model is trained to establish w and b.

Vectors x_i for which $|y_i|(wx_i^T + b) = 1$ will be termed support vector (Figure 4.1). As a linear classifier, the SVM method was originally developed by Vapnik (7) in 1963. It is also possible to model non-linear, high-dimensional models using SVM using the kernel technique (8). The application of a kernel function to increase the dimensions of the raw data can result in the linearization of a non-linear problem in a higher-dimensional space. A kernel function may be able to speed up some calculations that would otherwise require calculations in high-dimensional space. According to its definition, it is as follows:

$$K(x, y) = < f(x), f(y) > \tag{4.5}$$

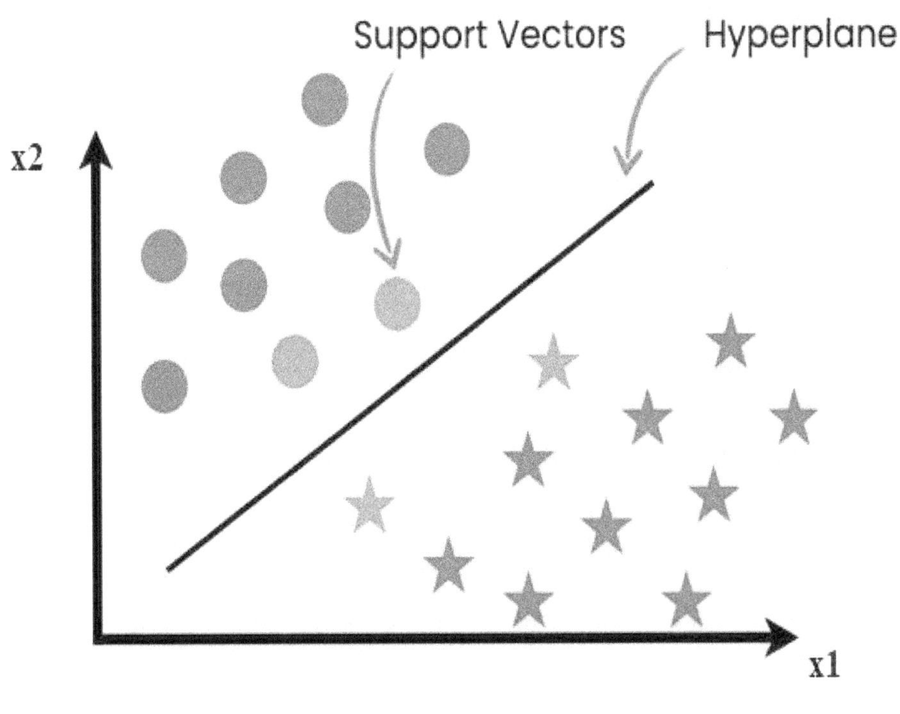

Figure 4.1 SVM model

4.4 ARTIFICIAL NEURAL NETWORK (ANN)

Neural Networks (ANNs) are a type of distributed computing influenced by biology. It consists of network connections and basic processing units, or nodes. One way to gauge how much one unit will influence another is to look at the weight of the connection between any two units. These nodes—which carry out thresholding and summation—are composed of two subsets of the units: input and output. To get over the over-fitting issue, an early halting method is typically employed. Using an independent validation set, the early halting technique monitors network performance. Typically, when a network adjusts to the unique characteristics of the training set, the validation set's errors first decrease and then increase.AI-based ANNs have been successfully used in a variety of fields, including network reliability, sports winning prediction, marketing, retail, financial services, insurance, telecommunications, and operations management (Smith & Gupta 2000, Srivarre-Ratana *et al.* 2022).

4.4.1 Learning of ANN

The network is trained by the ANN through a learning process. Weights are changed during training to get the required amounts. Supervised and unsupervised learning are the two main categories into which the learning can be divided. It involves the provision of examples of inputs and outputs as inputs to supervised learning. In order to lower the error between the output of the network and the actual output, the weights are adjusted. When building the training set, extra care must be used. A training set that accurately reflects the underlying model is the ideal. A highly dependable and comprehensive model cannot be generated from an unrepresentative training set. The network needs to be trained before it can use supervised learning. A network may be put into operation once the weights have been fixed for the outputs that result from a set of inputs. Unsupervised learning, however, does not use training set output values as target values. The network looks only at the input data to find the underlying pattern or trend. Different learning procedures are needed for different kinds of networks. For ANNs to accomplish various learning objectives, a wide variety of learning schemes have been developed. The learning strategies that are most commonly employed include nearest neighbour and error correction techniques.

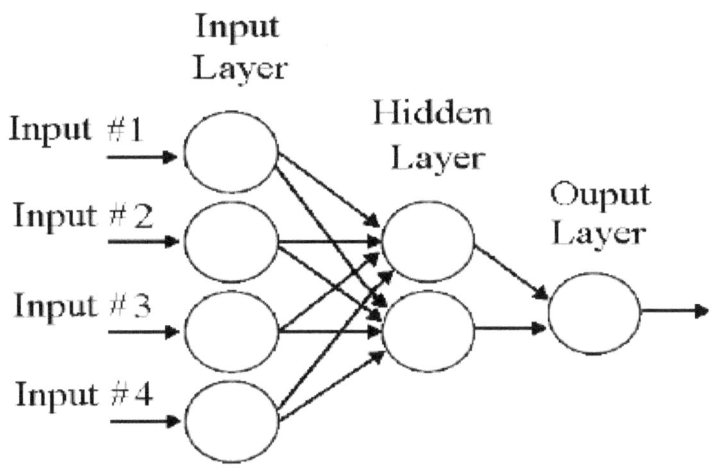

Figure 4.2 General topology of ANN

From the huge amount of study on computers, a novel idea that has emerged is the potential to simulate the brain's processing mechanism. In terms of recognition, analysis, prediction, and even learning, the biological unit still outperforms any artificial instrument, but the appealing performance of the brain-simulation models has generated sufficient motivation for additional research. The brain's highly networked structure serves as the foundation for the ANN method. This method outperforms its traditional counterparts in terms of speed, robustness in noisy settings, problem-solving flexibility, and great adaptability to novel contexts. Owing to these well-established benefits, the ANN is being used in many real-world applications, including robotics, speech recognition, image processing, and stock market forecasting. Its application in system engineering-related domains like rainfall-runoff modelling, rule-based control, and time series prediction has been the subject of substantial research.

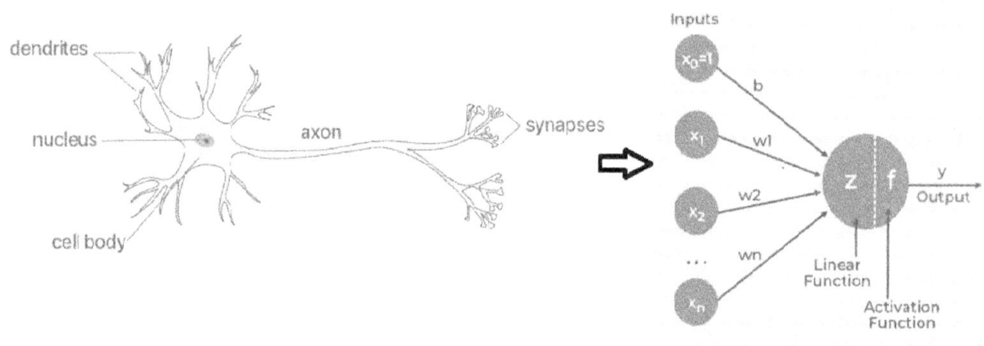

Figure 4.3 Biological and Artificial Neural Networks

The forward and backward passes are the two steps of a feed-forward neural network. After receiving a sample input, activations are passed through the network until they reach the output layer. There are several common activation functions, including linear sum, sigmoid, and Gaussian functions. By comparing the actual output with the intended output, backward error estimates are calculated for the output units. To reduce errors, it may be necessary to adjust the weights associated with output units.

4.5 RANDOM FOREST (RF)

Inspired by earlier research by Amit & Geman (1997), Breiman (2001) introduced Random Forests. Random Forests, which were created as an alternative to boosting, are extensions of Breiman's bagging concept (Breiman 2001), despite the description in that work making this clear. In Breiman (2001), Random Forests can be used to analyze either categorical or continuous response variables (called classification or regression, respectively). Similar to this, categorical or continuous predictor variables are also possibilities. The procedures for building decision trees are provided by the Random Forest Algorithm (Dietterich 2000) below.

- Assume that the samples contain N occurrences of the training data. Assume that the input dataset has M attributes.
- A minimum of m parameters should be provided in the input to determine which attribute will be selected next at each node in the tree (where m is less than M). Each sample is replaced with a replacement tree once the training samples have been collected.
- In each node of the tree, choose m attributes at random.
- The sample dataset's m input attributes are used to calculate the optimal split.
- Every tree is grown without any pruning.

4.5.1 Merits of Random Forest Algorithm

- Accuracy is superior.
- Skilled in managing huge databases.
- Handles thousands of input variables quickly and easily.
- Offers details on significant variables that are not included in the classification.
- Offers techniques for approximating absent information.
- Maintains missing data without sacrificing accuracy.
- Information or Meta data regarding the relationships between various variables are provided by prototypes.
- Permits the investigation of variable interactions.

4.5.2 Random Forest Applications

Banking: To identify devoted clients and fraudulent clients, a random forest algorithm is employed in this industry. Additionally, it helps bankers identify clients who might not be profitable for the institution. Moreover, arbitrators and defaulters might be identified by organizations.

Medicine: The random forest algorithm is frequently used in the medical field to determine the best possible combination of symptoms and disease-related elements. Analysing the patient's medical records does this.

Stock Market: The behaviour of stock movements and the anticipated profit or loss for buying a specific stock is determined using the Random Forest algorithm.

E-commerce: Customer segmentation is the process of identifying purchase trends and forecasting more similar types of consumers.

4.5.3 Limitations of Random Forest Model

- One of the most common issues in the literature, particularly with regression tasks, is over-fitting to a specific data sample (Louppe 2014).
- Random forests struggle to manage properties with multiple values and dimensions. They prefer multi-level categorical variables (Jampani *et al.* 2015).

In Random Forests, trees $h_j(X,\theta_j)$ are used as base learners. A fitted tree is known as $\hat{h}_j(x,\theta_j,D)$ for a particular realization of θ_j of θ_j, when $D=\{(x_1,y_1),\ldots(x_N,y_N)\}$, and $x_i=(x_{i,1},\ldots\ldots,x_{i,p})^T$ represents the p predictors and yi represents the response.

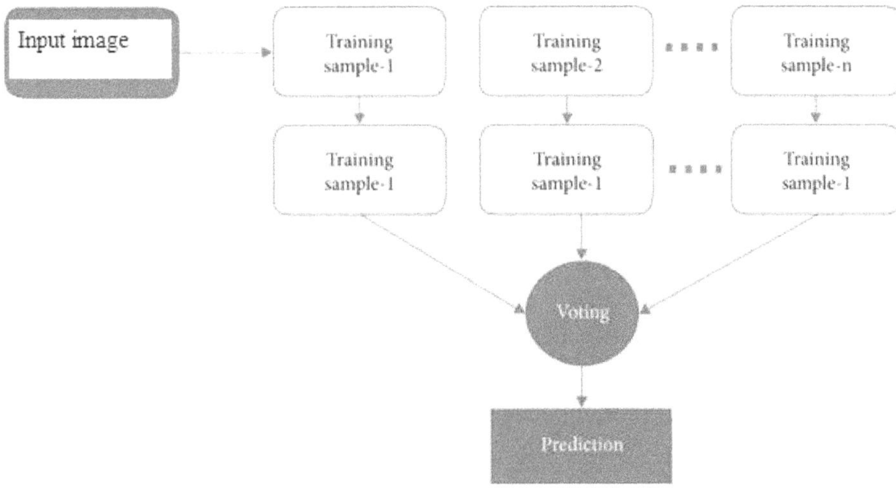

Figure 4.4 Random forest algorithm

The random component θ_j is not explicitly considered by Breiman in his original formulation (Hrehorow *et al.* 2012) but is implicitly used to generate unpredictability in two ways. A bootstrap sample is first taken from the original data to fit each tree, as in the case of bagging. A portion of θ_j is provided by randomization in bootstrap sampling. A second difference is that when splitting a node, an optimal split is chosen using a random subset of m predictor variables rather than an individual split for each of the p predictor variables. As a result of the randomization in which the predictors are sampled, the remaining component of θ_j is determined. During the maturation process, the trees are not pruned.

It was initially suggested by Hrehorow et al. (2012) to grow them until the terminal nodes were pure (classification), or they contained no more than a predetermined number of data points (regression). A limit on the number of terminal nodes is suggested by Segal & Xiao (2011). Whenever categorical responses are produced (classification), they are blended using unweighted voting; when continuous responses are produced (regression), they are averaged using unweighted averaging.

4.6 PROPOSED METHODOLOGY

Algorithm 4.3: Random Forests

Input: Pre-processed input images

Output: Segmented output images

Let $D = \{(x_1, y_1), .. (x_N, y_N)\}$, denote the training data, with $x_i = (x_{i,1}, ..., x_{i,p})^T$.

For $j = 1$ to J

1. Take a bootstrap sample D_j of size N from D

2. Using the bootstrap sample D_j as the training data, fit a tree using binary recursive partitioning

a. Start with all observations in a single node.

b. Repeat the following steps recursively for each unsplit node until the stopping criterion is met:

i. Select m predictors at random from the p available predictors.

ii. Find the best binary split among all binary splits on the m predictors from step i.

iii. Split the node into two descendant nodes using the split from step

To make a prediction at a new point x,

$$\hat{f}(x) = \frac{1}{j} \sum_{j=1}^{J} I\left(h_j x( ) = y\right)$$ for classification

4.7 AUTOMATIC SEGMENTATION OF PSORIASIS SKIN IMAGES USING ACHOA BASED CNN

4.7.1 Overview

An outline of the proposed model for psoriasis skin image segmentation can be seen in Figure 4.5. In order to segment psoriasis skin images, training images are resized and pixel values are scaled between zero and one. Next, the segmentation model is applied to the preprocessed images. We present a CNN model based on AChOA that can be used to segment skin images with psoriasis. The segmentation model improves CNN performance by optimizing CNN's weight and bias settings using AChOA. A chaotic sequence based on a tent map is provided in order to improve the search performance of the ChOA method. As a result of the AChOA-CNN structure, probability maps are produced. Using a thresholding module, a binary mask is then created based on the proposed model. The segmented output's undesired artefacts will be eliminated in this module.

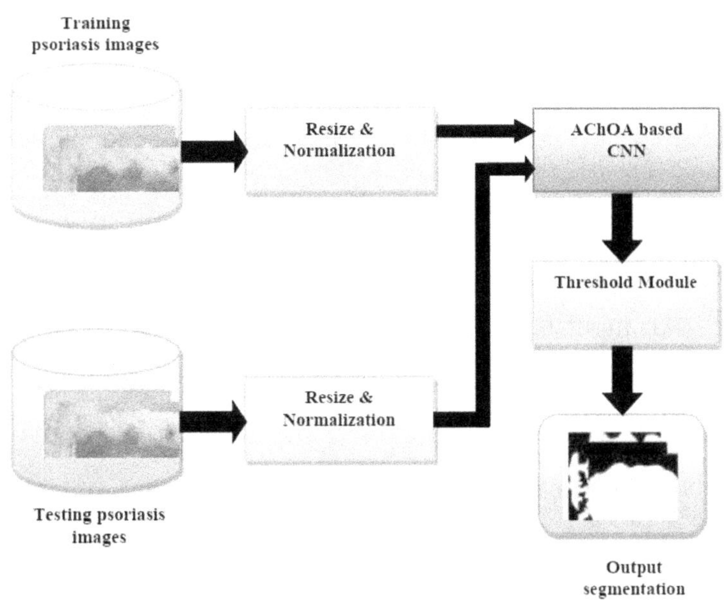

Figure 4.5 Structure of the proposed psoriasis segmentation model

4.7.2 Materials and Methods

A dataset of psoriasis skin images is gathered from private clinical practices. A total of 8000 skin images are included in this data collection. The total number of images consists of 4200 images depicting skin with psoriasis, and 3800 images showing healthy skin. The human body parts depicted in these skin photos include the mouth, chest, palm, and hand, among others. A resolution other than 640x480 may be present in the images. Six, 400 of the total images are used for training purposes, and 1,600 are used for testing purposes. About 48 percent of the photographs in this collection are Asian, 22 percent are Black, 12 percent are Hispanic, and 18 percent are Caucasian. There are also 646 mild images, 1207 moderate images, 1271 severe images, and 1076 extremely awful images.

4.7.3 Training Phase

The suggested segmentation model was trained using 80 percent of the dataset's images of psoriasis skin. Prior to segmenting the input images, each image's size is adjusted, and each pixel's value is scaled between 0 and 1. The suggested AChOA-based CNN is then trained with the pre-processed images to identify the psoriasis region. The following sections provide an explanation of how the suggested segmentation model is implemented.

4.7.4 CNN

An input layer, a convolutional layer, and a pooling layer are the three layers of the proposed CNN's layered architecture. Layers are grouped according to their relative importance, and a FCL follows. In order to exclude undesirable pixels from the input image, this proposed system first filters it in the convolutional layer. After the convolutional layer, the output is fed into the maximum pooling layer. By using this layer, the dimensions of the feature are reduced without affecting their characteristics. The following describes how each layer in the CNN architecture functions.

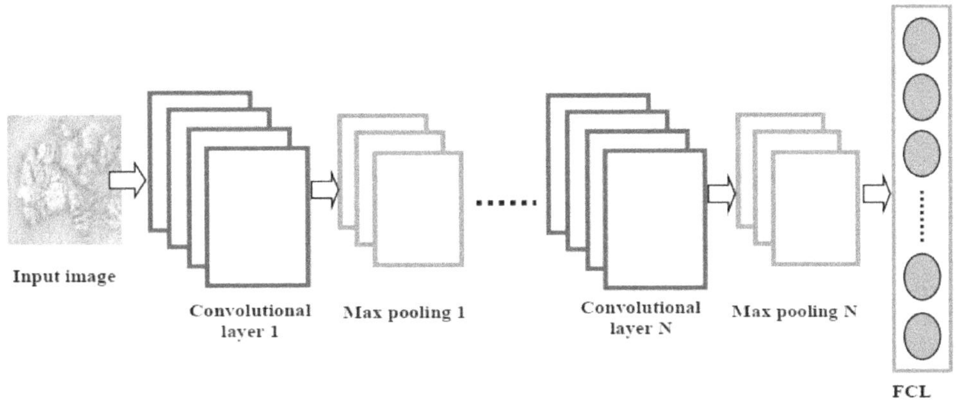

Figure 4.6 Structure of CNN

Convolutional layer: The convolutional layer is the most important layer in the CNN structure. In this case, the conversion matrix is used to generate the feature change map. Using this method, the filter size is assumed to be 5 by 5, as opposed to the more commonly used 3 by 3 or 5 by 5. Using the change layer as an example, the following equation can be used to represent the output.

$$B_i^b = \sum_{j \in F_i} B_j^{b-1} \otimes \xi_{ij}^b + L_i^b \tag{4.6}$$

where, $\otimes$ represents the Convolution operator, ξ^b_{ij} representsthe Weight value for the ith filter for the bth convolutional layer, L^b_i represents the Bias of the ith filter of the bth convolutional layer and B_i^b is the Activation map.

Pooling layer: CNN's tier-based structure includes the pooling layer following the convolutional layer. Its planes are the same as the conventional layer's. The computational load on the network is reduced by this layer by reducing the spatial dimensions of the feature map. Each feature map is subject to a different pooling layer. The maximum pooling method and the average pooling method are two popular methods for pooling. With maximum pooling, the abstract format of the original image remains while the average pooling images are balanced and it becomes more difficult to distinguish the image's clear features. Maximum pooling outperforms average pooling layer when it comes to image data. It is therefore recommended to employ the largest pooling layer in the recommended method. In this case, the image is divided into two equal matrices of volume. Pool feature maps are produced by transferring the F-size feature map over the pooling layer during peak pooling operations. As shown in equation (4.7), the pooling map represents the pooling process.

$$P_i = \underset{j \in R_j}{Max}\, F_i \tag{4.7}$$

Fully connected layer (FCL): The (FCL) is comprised of a feed-forward neural network. Maximum attached layer receives its input from the maximum pooling layer. The selected features are supplied to the detection level by a software function at the end of the release. The input image consists of three layers that are fully integrated and five transition layers. In order to generate rear probability scores, the Softmax layers separate the temporal and spatial aspects of the image. For further processing, we use the resulting probability map.

4.7.5 Psoriasis Skin Images Segmentation using AChOA based CNN

The purpose of this section is to describe the process by which the AChOA algorithm achieves the ideal CNN weights and bias values. The term "chimps" has been used in ChOA [92] for chimpanzees. There is the greatest similarity between chimpanzees and humans in terms of the Brain to Body Ratio (BBR). The greater the BBR of mammals, the greater the level of intelligence. In addition to sharing the same DNA, humans and chimpanzees are both descended from ancient hominoid creatures. Chimpanzee colonies fluctuate in size due to changes in time and member movement within their natural habitat, as they typically belong to a fission-fusion society. Using a method unique to itself, each colony group autonomously finds the hunt space. Chimpanzees hunt on their own in all groups. Everybody's skills come in handy in any circumstance.

In addition, the colony is home to four different species of chimps, which include:

- Drivers: A driver does not attempt to capture its prey; instead, he follows it.
- Barriers: They ensconce themselves in trees in order to extend their dam across the movement of their prey.
- Chasers: In order to catch their prey, they pursue them swiftly
- Attackers: The breaking path of the prey is calculated in order to rehunt or drive the prey to the shelter below.

Chimpanzee hunting typically consists of two main stages: "exploration," which includes driving, obstructing, and pursuing the prey (see Figure 4.7), and "exploitation," which includes attacking the victim (see Figure 4.8). The numbers in question have been adjusted from (Khishe Mohammad & Mohammad RezaMosavi 2020).

A chaotic sequence based on a tent map is also incorporated in this study in order to enhance the initial quality of the population and the capability of ChOA to carry out searches. A deterministic framework can also be chaotic. There are numerous map functions used for chaotic framework. Among them, logistic maps and tent maps are frequently utilised. However, as the tent map function has more uniform features and the logistic map has unequal traversal characteristics, it is used in this work.

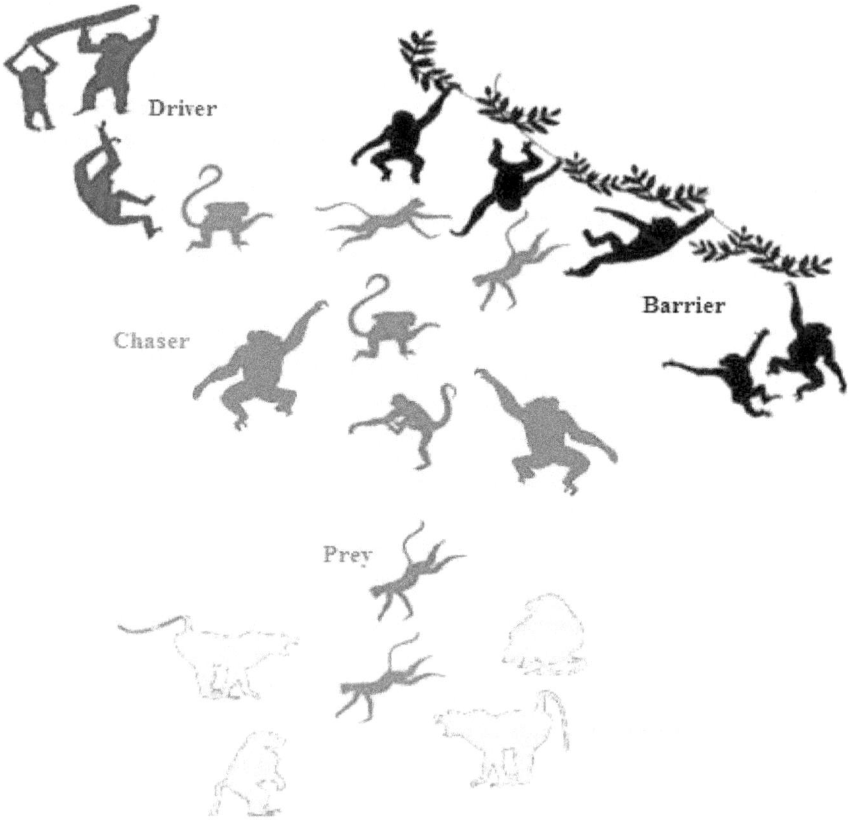

Figure 4.7 Exploration process

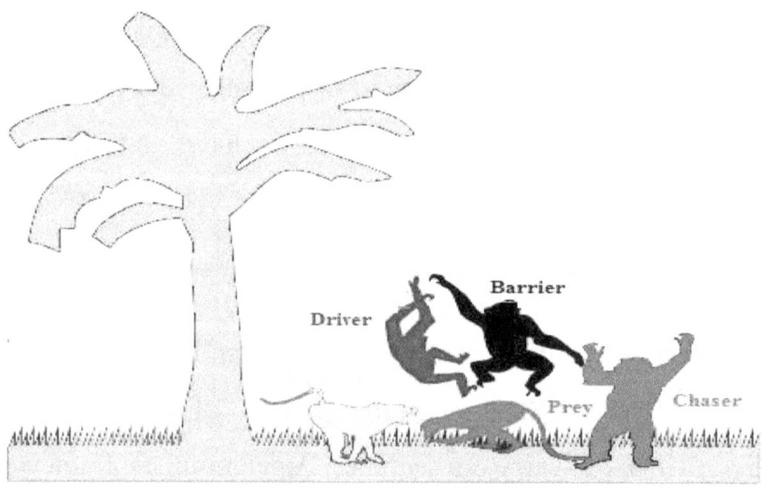

Figure 4.8 Exploitation process

Using AChOA's optimal path selection algorithm, the following steps are taken:

Initialization: This algorithm involves a chimp relating the solution to another chimp. CNN parameters, like bias (L) and weight (ξ), are used as solutions. (4.8) is used to define the population's initialization.

$$P_N = \{y_1, y_2, \ldots, y_N\} \tag{4.8}$$

where, y_N represents the Nth solution and it is depicted using (4.9).

$$y_N = \{\xi_1, \xi_2, \ldots, \xi_i; L_1, L_2, \ldots, L_i\} \tag{4.9}$$

Chaotic sequence based on tent map: A description of the function of the tent map can be found in equation (4.10).

$$q^{k+1} = \begin{cases} q_k / a & q_k < a \\ (1-q_k)/(1-a) & q_k \geq a \end{cases} \tag{4.10}$$

There is a random initial value for q_k within the range [0, 1] which represents the chaotic sequence. *Here, a is fixed as 0.7, which denotes the control parameter for the fractal.* A chaotic sequence $\{q_1, q_2, \ldots\ldots q_m\}$ is generated for each iteration using (4.10). By using (4.11), we are able to map the sequence to the first solution.

$$\left({}_{d} \quad {}_{d,\min} \right) {}_{d,\max} \quad + {}_{d,\min} \quad {}_{d} \tag{4.11}$$

Here, $y_{d,\min}$ and $y_{d,\max}$ denote the lower boundary and upper boundary of y in the dth dimension respectively. During initialization, chaotic population is generated by mapping the solutions in the population using (4.10) and (4.11).

Objective function (fitness) calculation: This method assesses fitness based on segmentation accuracy. The definition of fitness calculation is as follows:

$$Fit_N = Max\,(Accuracy) \tag{4.12}$$

The accuracy can be determined as follows,

$$Accuracy = \frac{TN + TP}{TP + FP + TN + FN} \tag{4.13}$$

Here, TP - true positive

FP- false positive

TN- true negative

FN- false negative

It can be concluded that the weight and bias values of the CNN that yield maximum fitness are considered the ideal parameters according to equation (4.12). The prey's state is here represented by the optimal solution state. The solution is modified in the following manner if the necessary fitness is not discovered.

Update the solution: In the following phases, we discuss how the chimps' hunting behavior can be expressed mathematically.

Driving and Chasing the Prey: We define these processes with the help of (4.14) and (4.15).

$$z = \left| y_{prey}(t) \times c - y_{chimp}(t) \times n \right| \tag{4.14}$$

$$y_{chimp}(t+1) = y_{prey}(t) - b \times z \tag{4.15}$$

Where, t -current iteration,

y_{prey}- prey's position

b, c and n- coefficient vectors

This vector of coefficients is defined in terms of (4.16), (4.17) and (4.18),

$$b = 2 \times f \times rand_1 - f \tag{4.16}$$

$$c = 2 \times rand_2 \tag{4.17}$$

$$n = Chaotic\_value \tag{4.18}$$

where, $rand_1$ and $rand_2$ are the random vectors [0, 1], f represents Coefficient vector which is reduced non-linearly from 2.5 down to 0 and n represents the chaotic vector, which shows how chimpanzee sexual arousal affects hunting performance, was computed using the difference chaotic map.

Exploitation or attacking stage: Attacking chimps often carry out the hunting process. The prey's location can be determined mathematically by comparing the best answers. The four best solutions that were found are combined. Subsequently, the remaining chimps' positions will be adjusted to match the top chimps' positions.

This phase is describe by (4.19), (4.20) and (4.21).

$$z_{Attacker} = |y_{Attacker} \times c_1 - y \times n_1|, \qquad z_{Barrier} = |y_{Barrier} \times c_2 - y \times n_2|$$

$$z_{Chaser} = |y_{Chaser} \times c_3 - y * n_3| \qquad z_{Driver} = |y_{Driver} \times c_4 - y \times n_4| \tag{4.19}$$

$$y_1 = y_{Attacker} - z_{Attacker} \times b_1 \qquad y_2 = y_{Barrier} - z_{Barrier} \times b_2$$

$$y_3 = y_{Chaser} - z_{Chaser} \times b_3 \qquad y_2 = y_{Driver} - z_{Driver} \times b_4 \tag{4.20}$$

$$y(t+1) = \frac{y_1 + y_2 + y_3 + y_4}{4} \tag{4.21}$$

Prey attacking stage: Here, the chimps attack the victim, and the hunting process ends when the creature stops moving. It is necessary to reduce the coefficient f value in this stage's mathematical equation. As well as lowering the value of f, lowering the value of b also has the effect of lowering its range. A significant change in the range of b occurs during iteration during the interval [-2f, 2f], in which the value of f falls from 2.5 to 0. Chimps select the next site between their present location and their prey's prior position when the value of b is between -1 and 1. Figure 4.9 from (Godin & Touitou 2007) illustrates the chimps striking a prey positioned as depicted in figure 4.9.

Exploration stage: Chimpanzees are compelled in this situation to leave their prey and go for better prey. If the value of b is more than 1 or less than -1, the chimps should split from the prey, according to the mathematical expression of divergence behaviour. This procedure makes the global search algorithm possible. Figure 4.9 illustrates the way in which chimpanzees search for their prey. As a result of this method, the local minimum is further avoided by using the c factor inside [0, 2]. Assigning a random weight to the prey is the function of this element.

Social motivation: At this point, chimps fulfil their hunting obligations due to their social motive. Then, in a much disorganised fashion, they attempt to obtain meat. In high-dimensional circumstances, chimpanzees are able to overcome the two problems of capturing in local optima and a slower rate of convergence due to their chaotic final stage behavior. In addition to enhancing the effectiveness of ChOA, chaotic maps have also been used to enhance its effectiveness. These chaotic maps behave like discrete fixed cycles. Using (17), this behaviour is defined.

$$y_{Chimp}(t+1)=\begin{cases} y_{prey}(t)-b\times z & if\ \eta < 0.5 \\ Chaotic\_value & if\ \eta > 0.5 \end{cases} \tag{4.22}$$

where, η - random number within [0, 1].

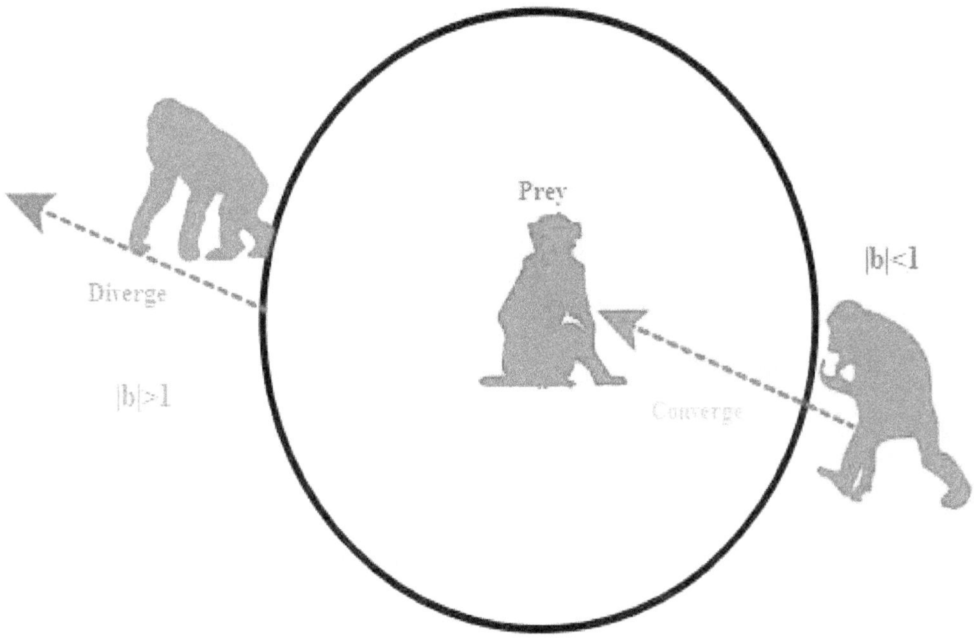

Figure 4.9 Chimps update the position depend on |b|

Termination: The solution is updated as soon as the weight and bias of CNN are determined. A solution is obtained at the end of the algorithm.

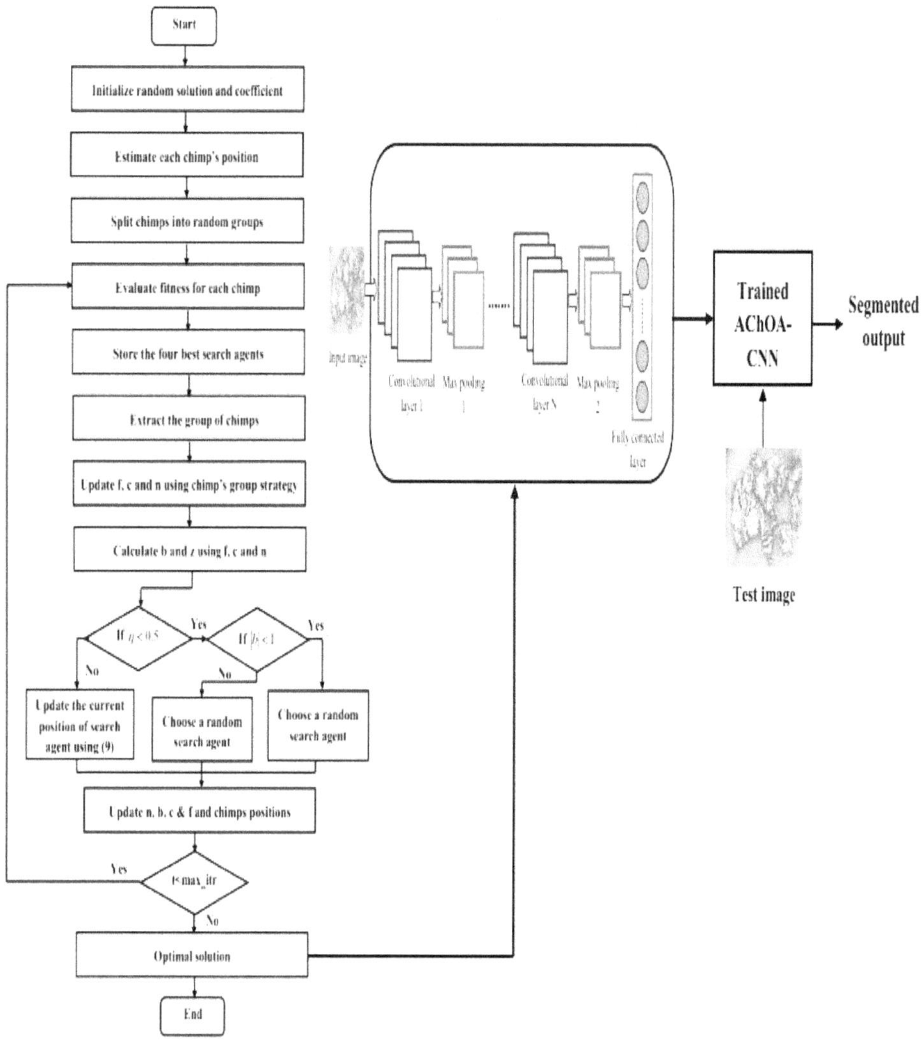

Figure 4.10 Training and Testing Phases of AChOA-CNN

4.7.6 Testing Phase

This phase involves scaling the images and normalizing their pixel values to fall between 0 and 1. A trained segmentation model is applied to the preprocessed test images after they have been preprocessed. A probability map illustrating the segmentation outcome is included in the output that results. '0' denotes normal skin in the segmented image, whereas '1' denotes the presence of an infected region.

4.7.8 Threshold Module

The probability map shows the likelihood that each pixel is related to either the surrounding skin or psoriasis. Following the acquisition of the probability map, a binary mask is obtained through the usage of the threshold module to facilitate further evaluation of the suggested model. Once the probability maps are seen and examined, the threshold value of 0.8 is fixed, providing an optimal binary mask. Equation (4.23), which describes the threshold module condition.

$$o/p = \begin{cases} 1 & \textit{if pixel value} \geq 0.8 \\ 0 & \textit{Otherwise} \end{cases} \tag{4.23}$$

We would like to inform you that there are less pixels included in the injuries (artefacts) than there are in the injuries themselves (psoriasis). Additionally, discrete areas have been drawn for every corresponding component, and images with a variety of related components have been selected. Smaller region components are removed after the pre-threshold, which is set at 600, is used to define the region for each designated associated portion. The output from the threshold module and the subsequent deformation removal from the resultant image are shown in Figure 4.11.

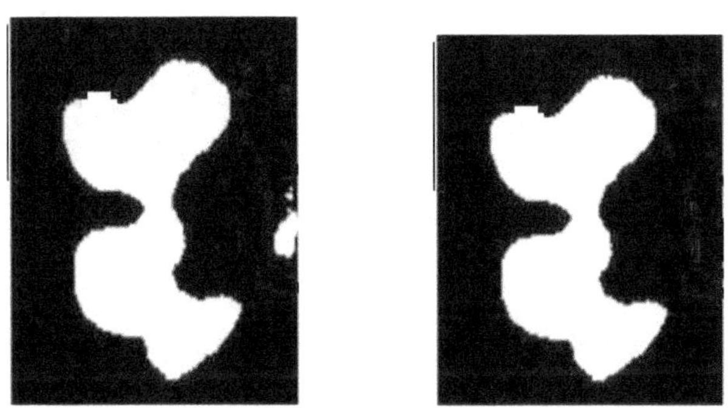

(a) **(b)**

Figure 4.11 (a) The Threshold module's output, (b) Artifacts removed from output

4.8 RESULTS AND DISCUSSIONS

A Windows 10 PC with a Core i3 processor and 4GB RAM is used to simulate the recommended segmentation model in MATLAB 2020a. Several private clinics provided images of psoriasis for this study. The input images are shown with the matching segmented outputs in Figure 4.12. During the simulation, the CNN model based on AChOA is trained using 80% of the images, with 20% set aside for testing the trainingmodel.

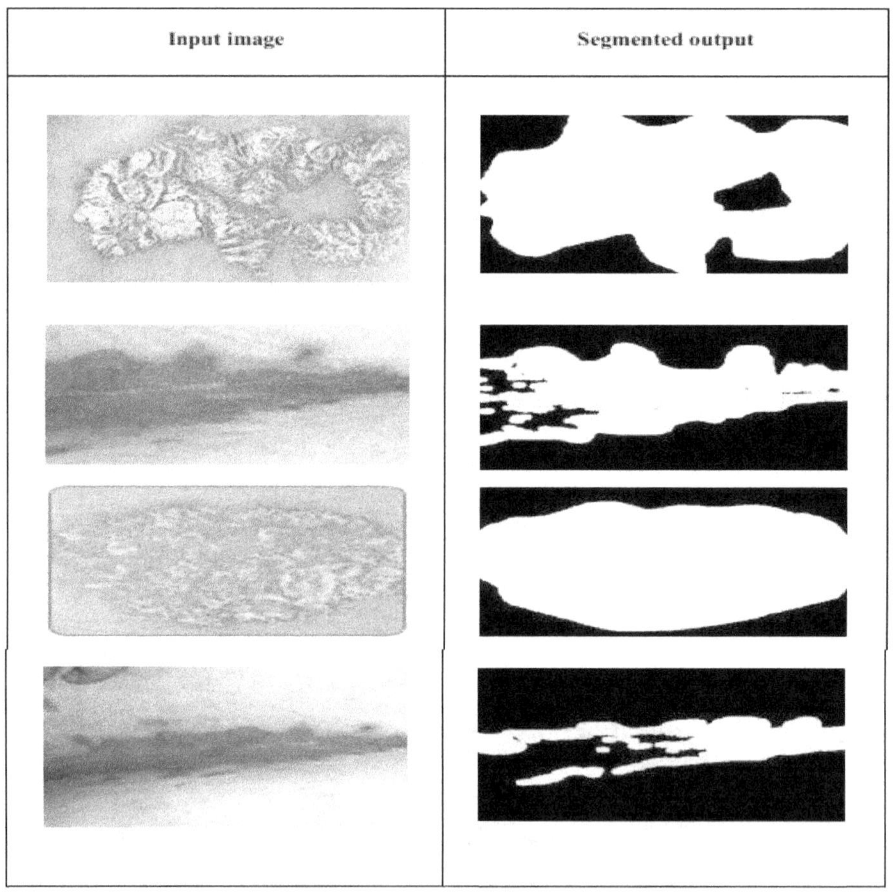

Figure 4.12 Input image and segmented output

The suggested CNN has two transposed convolution layers, one max pooling layer, twenty-nine convolution layers, twenty-four ReLU layers, and twenty-six batch normalisation layers in the simulation. Additionally, a performance comparison is made between AChOA-CNN and other segmentation models that are currently in use, including CNN, SVM, ANN, and random forest (RF).

4.9 EVALUATION OF METRICS

A segmentation model's performance is evaluated using the following metrics.

- *Accuracy*: Equation (4.13) already expresses its use in computing the input image's accurate segmentation rate.
- *Sensitivity*: Equation (4.24) defines its use: it is utilised to precisely segment the affected region in the images.

$$Sensitivity = \frac{TP}{FN + TP} \tag{4.24}$$

- *Specificity*: Equation (4.25) defines it, and it's utilised to precisely segment the non-infected area in the images.

$$Specificity = \frac{TN}{FP + TN} \tag{4.25}$$

- *Jaccard index*: It is employed to quantify the shift in the image axis's centre of infection.

$$JI = \frac{TP}{FP + FN + TP} \tag{4.26}$$

- *Dice coefficient:* In this method, a binary label is compared with the image's predictions in order to calculate the ratio.

$$DC = \frac{2TP}{FP + FN + 2TP} \tag{4.27}$$

4.10 PERFORMANCE ANALYSIS

This section compares and evaluates the segmentation models' accuracy, sensitivity, specificity, JI, and DC. The accuracy comparison of several segmentation models is displayed in Figure 4.13. With an accuracy of 94%, the CNN-based segmentation model beat SVM, ANN, and RF, as can be seen in the image. Even with only 18% Caucasian photos in the dataset, AChOA-CNN was able to increase its accuracy by 97% when the weight and bias parameters of the convolutional layer were optimized using AChOA. According to Figure 4.14, a sensitivity analysis of the segmentation model has been conducted. Based on the experimental results, the segmentation models currently employed - NNC, SVM, ANN, and RF - were capable of achieving sensitivity values of 95%, 92%, 91%, and 51%, respectively. It is noteworthy that this proposed AChOA-CNN segmentation model achieved a sensitivity of 98%, which is significantly higher than any other segmentation technique. Figure 4.15 illustrates the specificities of the various segmentation models. CNN-based segmentation achieved 99% specificity when compared to SVM, ANN, and RF. A chart illustrating the Jaccard index for each segmentation model can be found in Figure 4.16. The AChOA algorithm facilitates the smooth operation of CNN. Accordingly, AChOA-CNN surpassed CNN by 90% in terms of JI. Figure 4.17 shows the dice coefficients for a variety of segmentation models. A chart shows that the segmentation models currently used, such as CNN, SVM, ANN, and RF, achieved DIs of 92.95%, 91.73%, 59.17%, and 72.12%, respectively. The suggested segmentation model based on AChOA-CNN acquired a Dice coefficient of 96%, which is higher than prior segmentation approaches. Figure 4.18 shows the processing times for several segmentation models. It is interesting to note that the SVM-based segmentation model displayed 36% faster processing times than the ANN and RF-based segmentation models, as shown in the image below. CNN, which is renowned for its automated functioning, attained a respectable processing duration in contrast to alternative machine learning methods. SVM, ANN, and RF, for instance, performed 19%, 48%, and 51% faster than CNN-based segmentation models. Based on the optimisation of weights and bias values with the use of AChOA, the recommended segmentation model outperforms the standard CNN in terms of processing time. Compared to the standard CNN-based segmentation model, the suggested AChOA-CNN model performs 53% faster. An overview of the performance of the different segmentation methods can be found in Table 4.1. According to this table, the AChOA-CNN-based segmentation system performs better than the current CNN, SVM, ANN, and RF segmentation systems, with accuracies of 94.52%, 90.75%, 79.99%, and 74.99%. With a sensitivity of 98% and a specificity of 99%, the AChOA-CNN outperforms existing models. In addition, the segmentation system based on AChOA-CNN achieves JI and DC values of 90.5% and 96%, respectively, in comparison to earlier models. It is interesting to note that the entire computation time of the segmentation model suggested is only 20 seconds. Besides, training and testing time of the proposed scheme are evaluated and tabulated in this table. As depicted in the table, training time of the proposed scheme is 13s and testing time is 7s. Compared to existing models, the proposed model achieved better training and testing time.

Table 4.1 Analyze the performance of different algorithms for segmentation

Metrics	AChOA-CNN	CNN	SVM	ANN	RF
Accuracy	97%	94.52%	90.75%	79.99%	74.99%
Sensitivity	98%	95%	91%	90.5%	51%
Specificity	99%	97%	95%	67%	49%
JI	90.5%	88%	84%	61.5%	55.5%
DC	96%	92.95%	90.73%,	59.17%	72.12%
Processing time (sec)	20	43	53.5	82.5	88
Training time (sec)	13	28	33.5	52.5	57
Testing time (sec)	7	15	20	30	31

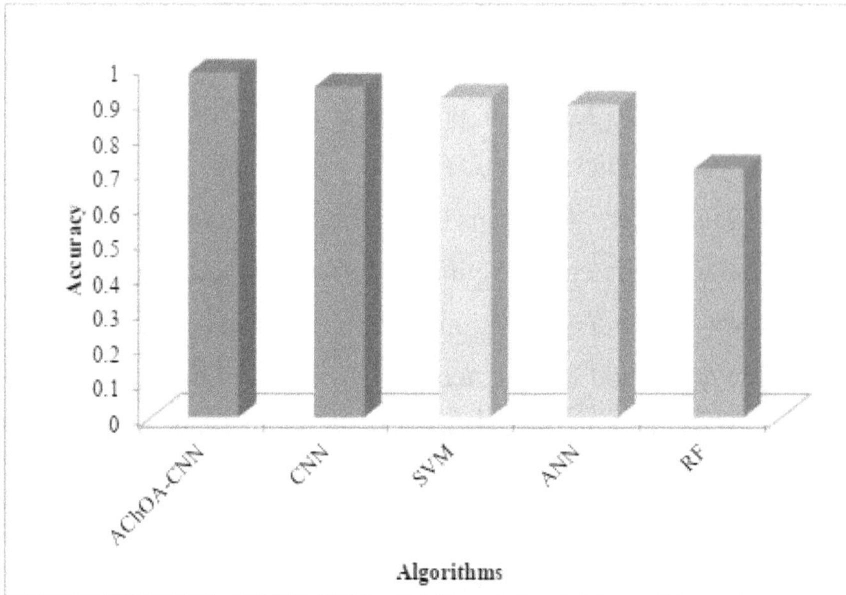

Figure 4.13 Accuracy of the different segmentation models

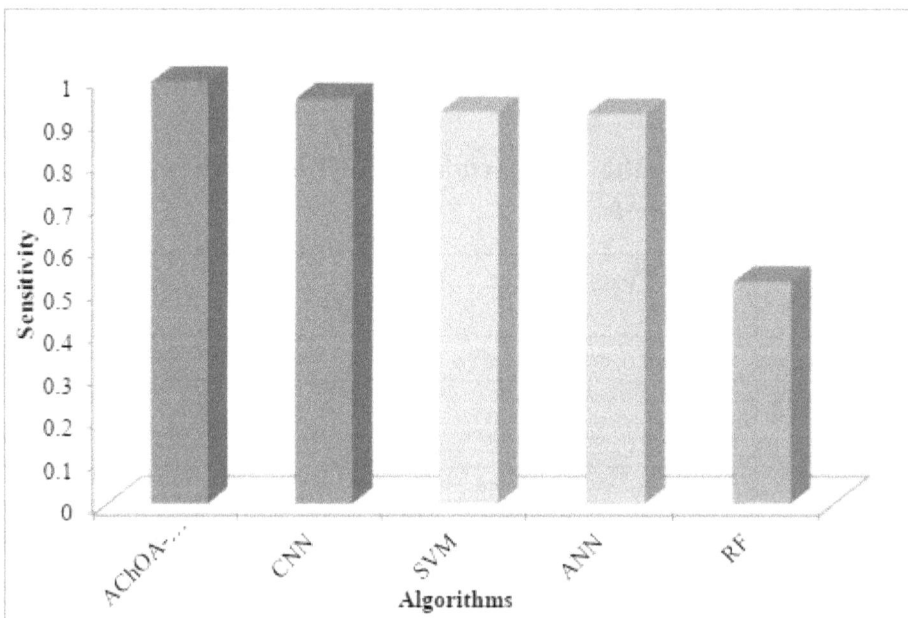

Figure 4.14 Sensitivity of the different segmentation models

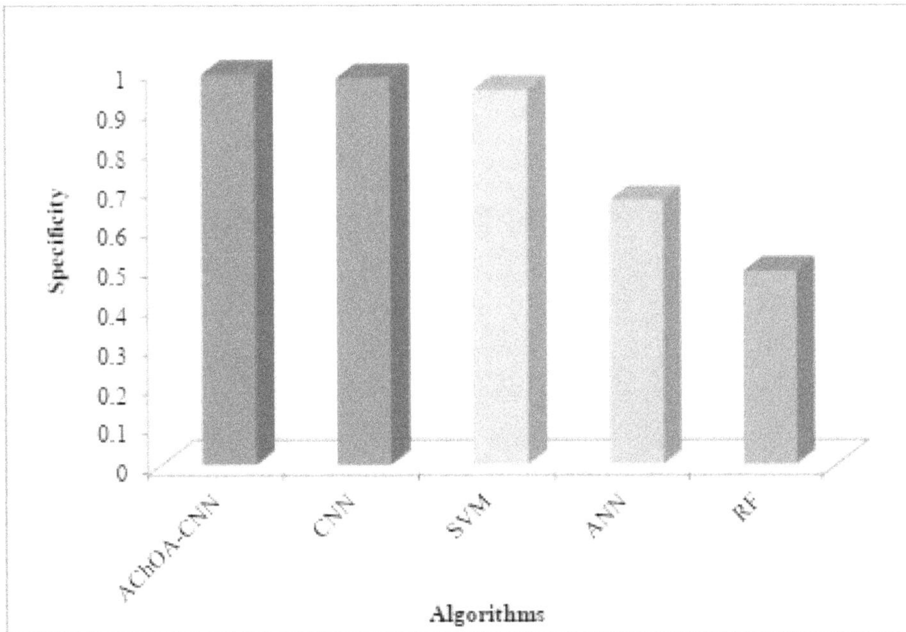

Figure 4.15 Specificity of the different segmentation models

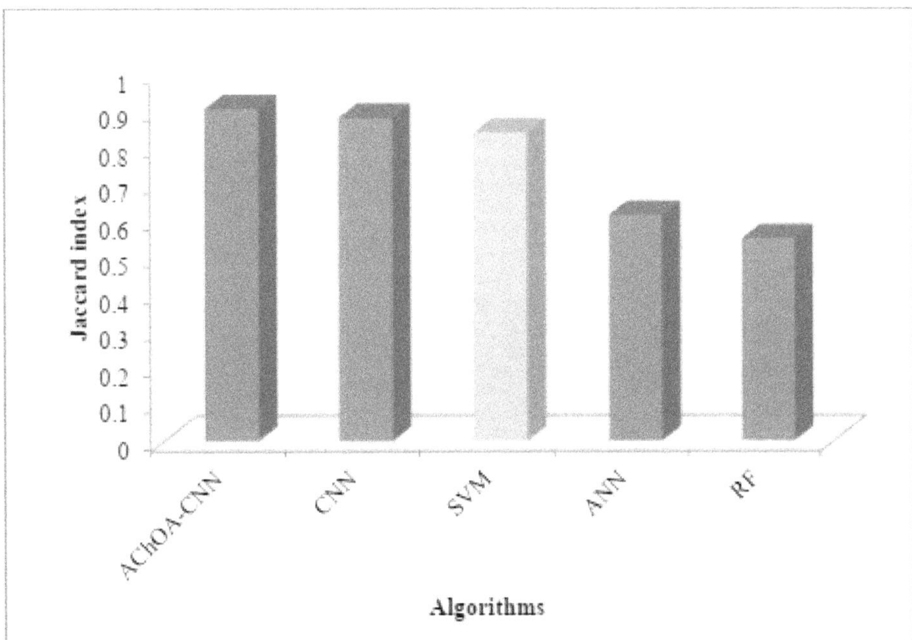

Figure 4.16 JI of the different segmentation models

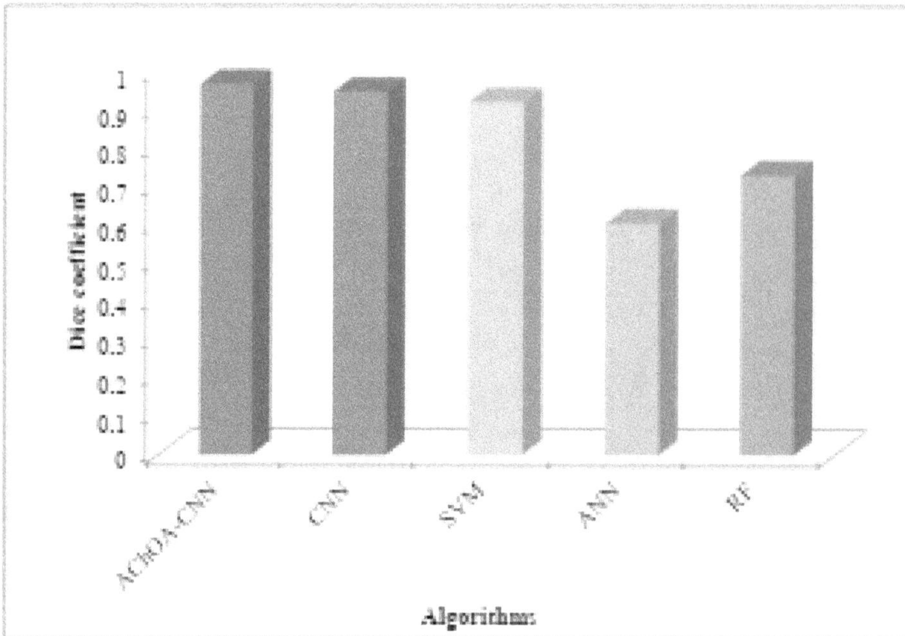

Figure 4.17 DC of the different segmentation models

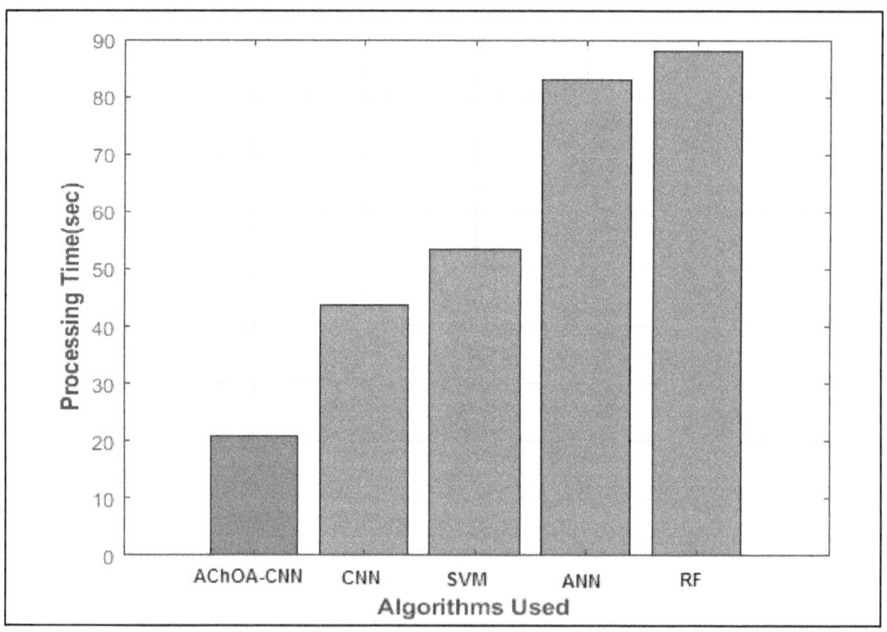

Figure 4.18 Processing time of different segmentation models

4.11 COMPARING THE PERFORMANCE OF THE PROPOSED METHOD WITH PREVIOUS LITERATURE

This division compares the proposed AChOA-CNN segmentation model's assessment criteria to those of earlier research. As shown in Table 4.2, the literatures (Dash *et al.* 2019, Raju *et al.* 2021, Arora *et al.* 2021, Dash *et al.* 2016, George *et al.* 2017, Griffiths *et al.* 2017) are taken into consideration for comparison. Londhe *et al.* demonstrated PsLSNet for psoriasis lesion segmentation (Dash *et al.* 2019). The data from the private clinic is used to assess the PsLSNet's performance. The inclusion of U shape in this model for feature extraction and contraction results in a minor increase in computing complexity. As a result, the accuracy drops to 2%. According to Raju *et al.* (2014), a combination of level set fuzzy c-means (FCM) algorithms has been devised for segmenting images of skin diseases. They evaluated the dataset derived from the ISIC-2018.Since CNN operates more effectively than FCM, the suggested scheme's accuracy is 5.4% higher than FCM's.

Arora *et al.* (2021) presented a technique for segmenting dermoscopic images using deep CNNs using attention. According to the authors, the ISIC-2018 dataset was used to evaluate attention-based deep CNNs. When the weights and bias parameters of the CNN are improved using AChOA, the proposed method is found to outperform the conventional deep CNN by 2% in accuracy. By Dash *et al.* (2020), a completely automated deep learning-based CADx algorithm for segmenting psoriasis photos has been developed. In the work, private clinical data were used. The writers segmented their data using U-Net. CNN has a lower computational complexity than U-Net. As a result, the suggested scheme's accuracy drops to 3.2%. The K-means algorithm was utilised by George Yasmeen and colleagues to segment psoriasis lesions. Among the other methods compared in the table, k-means clustering algorithm (2017) achieved the lowest accuracy.

Table 4.2 Evaluation of existing literatures with the suggested model

Ref	Dataset	Methods	Accuracy	Sensitivity	Specificity	JI	DC
Gelfand & Yeung (2012)	Private clinical Data	PsLSNet	0.951	0.905	0.988	0.880	0.933
Kimball *et al.*(2008)	ISIC-2018	Combination of the level set fuzzy c-means (FCM)	0.924	0.783	0.905	-	-
Love *et al.*(2011)	ISIC 2018	Attention-based deep CNN	0.952	0.913	0.972	0.864	0.921
El-Darouti & Hay (2010)	Private clinical Data	Fully automated deep learning-based CADx system	0.942	0.974	0.894	0.856	0.924
Randal Wickett & Marty Visscher (2006)	Private clinical Data	K-means algorithm	0.872	82.233	0.955	0.710	0.783
Proposed	**Private clinical Data**	**AChOA-CNN**	**0.971**	**0.984**	**0.995**	**0.900**	**0.963**

4.12 SUMMARY

The AChOA-CNN-based segmentation model is evaluated and simulated across a diverse range of images to raise the accuracy of psoriasis skin image segmentation. The pre-processing stage involves applying scaling and normalisation to the input psoriasis photos. The convolutional layer's weight and bias parameters are optimised by the augmented CNN using the pre-processed images and the AChOA method. The ChOA approach is further enhanced by incorporating a chaotic sequence based on a tent map in order to enhance search performance. Using the threshold module, artefacts from the segmented images are eliminated. The recommended segmentation model's performance is compared with segmentation models based on CNN, SVM, ANN, and RF. As per the study's conclusions, the suggested segmentation model based on AChOA-CNN attains 97% accuracy, 90% Jaccard Index (JI), and 96% Dice Coefficient (DC).

CHAPTER 5

AN EFFICIENT AUTOMATIC PSORIASIS DISEASE CLASSIFICATION USING DOUBLE-PATHWAY CASCADED CONVOLUTION NEURAL NETWORK

5.1 INTRODUCTION

The most prevalent type of the condition is chronic plaque psoriasis that is characterized by the growth of distinct red, scaly plaques in numerous sites on the body. (Griffiths *et al.* 2007). Early diagnosis reduces the risk of serious infection in the human body. Manual detection needs merely looking at the surface of the skin for the disease, which has certain disadvantages, such as human eyesight being incorrect, repeatable, and not quantitative. Despite the fact that skin infections are less lethal than other illnesses, they have a greater negative impact on quality of life due to the discomfort, stinging, and itching they cause. It is frequently afflicted by both common and rare illnesses.

5.2 METHODOLOGY

As a result, identifying human skin disorders is a difficult and ambiguous science. It has been highlighted that the majority of cases go undetected due to a lack of proper medical infrastructure and services. Early identification reduces the severity of illness in the human body. As a result, this research proposes automated psoriasis illness categorization using a Double-pathway cascaded convolution neural network (DPCCNN). In order to distinguish between a normal image and one with psoriasis, this research examines the DPCCNN with a single-pathway CNN that simultaneously extracts local and global properties. It is investigated in this study whether a cascaded CNN architecture can be used, by which the output of one CNN can be used as an additional input to succeeding CNNs. Adaptive Crocodile Optimization (ACO) is used to improve the classification performance of the fully connected layer by selecting the appropriate weight values. The first stages before categorization are pre-processing and image augmentation. Images are classed as normal or psoriatic images during the categorization step. Using the proposed approach, the experiment shows that it outperforms existing algorithms, including the most recent state-of-the-art approaches, achieving classification accuracy of over 96.5%.

5.3 EXISTING METHODOLOGY FOR PSORIASIS DISEASE CLASSIFICATION

5.3.1 Convolutional Neural Network (CNN)

In the field of artificial neural networks (ANNs), convolutional neural networks, also known as ConvNets, are characterized by their deep feed-forward architecture as well as their excellent generalization properties. It can detect and learn highly abstracted elements of things, particularly geographical data, more precisely than other networks with FC layers.

A deep CNN model consists of a few processing layers that can be taught to detect different features at different levels of abstraction from input data (like images). Higher abstraction is achieved by the deeper layers in learning and extracting low-level features, whereas lower-level features are learned and extracted by the initiatory levels.

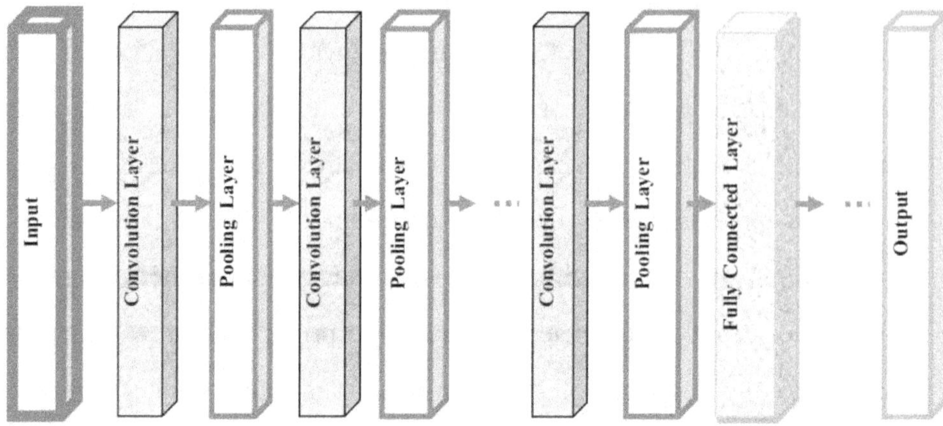

Figure 5.1 Conceptual model of CNN

Figure 5.1 breaks down the fundamental operation of the CNN example into four main components.

1. As with other types of ANNs, the input layer contains the pixel values of the image.

2. By calculating the scalar product between the weights of the neurons and the area associated with the input volume, the convolutional layer determines the output of neurons associated with certain local sections of the input. The rectified linear unit, or ReLU, is applied to the output of the activation produced by the previous layer in convolutional neural networks.

3. In the following step, the pooling layers will only downscale the input along its spatial dimensions, resulting in an activation with even fewer parameters.

4. The fully-connected layers will perform the tasks associated with conventional artificial neural networks and will generate

class scores based on the activations. Utilizing ReLu as a performance enhancer in between these layers is also advised.

5.3.1.1 Working principle of convolution neural network

Among its many uses are object identification, image classification, and medical image analysis. CNN is a multi-layer perception. The convolutional layer, polling layer, and fully connected layer are the three primary layers of CNN. Every layer has performed a different operation. Each layer performance is explained below;

Convolution layer: -The feature map is created with this layer. Here, we automatically extract the features of input image. In l^{th} layer, j^{th} feature map $\left(Y_j^{\,l}\right)$ is represented as follows;

$$Y_j^{\,l} = b_j^l + \sum_{i=1}^{in} k_{ji}^{\,l} * x_i^{l-1} \tag{5.1}$$

In this equation, b represents the bias value, j represents the index of the input channel, i represents the index of the output channel, and ***in*** indicates the total number of the feature maps. K represents the kernel weights and the prior layer feature map is given x_i^{l-1} and * depicts the convolution operator. In the frequency domain, convolution is the same as element-wise multiplication. So in Equation 5.1, is evaluated as $f^{-1}\{f\{k\}_i\{f(x)\}_i$, where, f indicates Fourier transform.

Pooling layer:- By using down-sampling, the pooling layer reduces the feature map. The down sampling expression is given in Equation (5.2).

$$PF = \left(F^E - P^O\right)/S + 1 \tag{5.2}$$

where, F^E represent the feature map size for before pooling.

Activation function: Activation functions are used to execute non-linear computations on datasets. Among the many different kinds of activation functions, rectifier linear unit (ReLU) activation functions, tangent, and sigmoid activation functions are often used in CNN-based algorithms to provide favorable results.

$$f(x) = \max(x,0) \tag{5.3}$$

Fully connected layer: At last, a completely connected layer converts labels and categories from high-level filtered images.

5.3.2 Single Path Cascaded CNN (SPCCNN)

Using a single pathway, the existing CNN architecture can assess patches with reduced kernel sizes, such as 33×33 and 5×5, and extract local characteristics from the impacted areas. This proposed CNN takes a 33 x 33 patch input as the first convolutional layer, and to incorporate the domain knowledge, it concatenates 5-batch features with the output feature maps of a second pooling layer. To improve segmentation performance, features need to be adapted to the proposed CNN architectures to determine more distinct boundaries between the impacted regions.

In spite of the fact that the proposed single-pathway CNN architecture with features is superior to existing single-path CNN-based approaches, it may not be appropriate for both local and global feature extraction from impacted regions. This is due to the nature of the affected regions. To address these problems, we also develop a cascaded CNN design using a single-pathway and different scales. Figure 5.2 illustrates this architecture, which combines the input of the second phase with the outputs of the first phase. In this architecture, two distinct patch types—53x53 and 33x33 with the same centre pixel—are employed to manage both local and global features. The first stage of the suggested single-pathway cascaded CNN processes the 53x53 patches and extracts the higher level properties. Processing 33×33 patches that are taken from the input images and the feature maps created by the previous phase is the aim of this second phase (Figure 5.2). Following their concatenation with the output feature maps of the second pooling layer of phase two, the feature-based patches pass through two convolutional layers. Here, the domain knowledge that improves the segmentation results is imposed by concatenating the feature-based patches to the second phase's intermediate layer. This architecture has an advantage over the single pathway CNN architecture for psoriatic image segmentation since it concentrates on both local and global attributes in addition to features.

The authors of Hussain *et al.* (2017) employed an incorrect patch size to determine the global and local features, despite the fact that their method similarly made use of cascaded CNN architecture. The authors (Hussain *et al.* 2017) employed comparatively bigger size kernels and an inadequate number of feature maps in order to extract the local features. However, Hussain *et al.* (2017) chose significantly smaller size patches, which had an impact on the effectiveness of their suggested strategy. With the help of various helpful features and patches and kernels of the right sizes, these kinds of weaknesses are addressed in the suggested cascaded CNN design. Furthermore, the suggested single-pathway cascaded CNN design outperforms the cascaded architecture in Ref. (Hussain et al. 2017) in terms of speed when the convolutional layer is substituted for the FCL in the last layer.

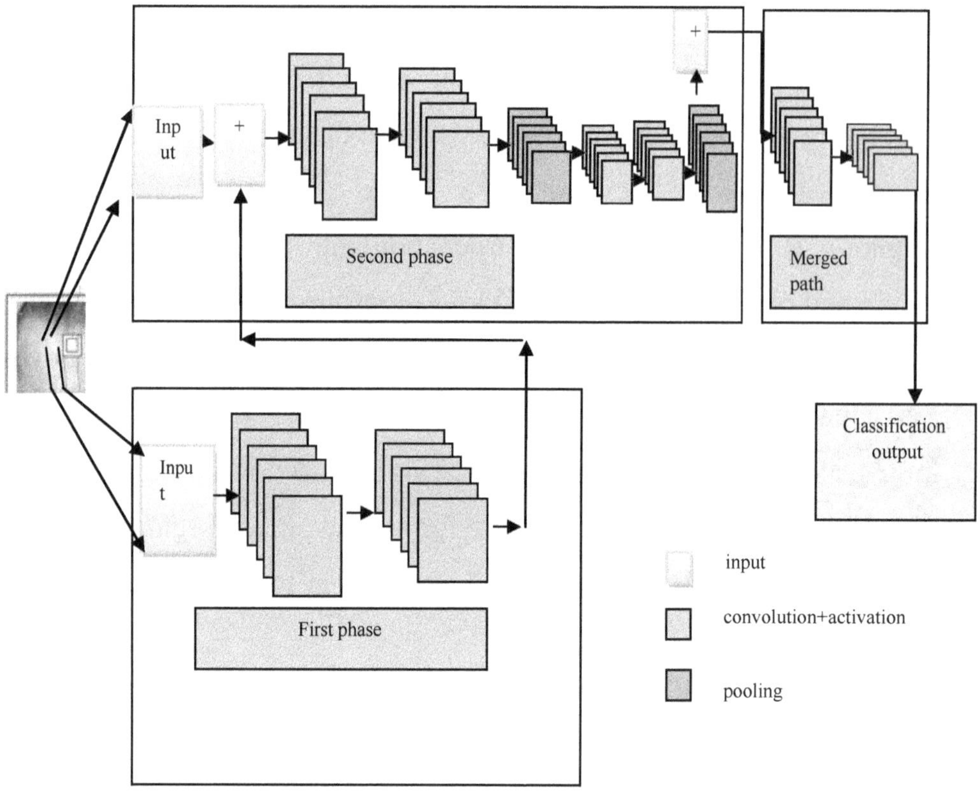

Figure 5.2 Single-Pathway Cascaded CNN

5.3.3 Deep Neural Network (DNN)

DNN architectures, in which the object is represented as primitives in layered composition, develop compositional models.

In comparison to a shallow network of equivalent efficiency, the extra layers enable the accumulation of components from lower levels, enabling the processing of huge amounts of data with fewer units. Information moves directly from the source to the target layers in DNNs. The great majority of DNN classifiers consist of structures with judgements based on the presumption that the amount of data in each category varies very minimally. When the influence of DNN climbs over a particular threshold, learning is modified in that classification group, and this results in a generalization effect.

It is possible to challenge the validity of non-homogeneous forms of case data. Given the foregoing, developing a DNN prediction approach is imperative. The effectiveness of the classifier's prediction is correlated with how challenging it is to remove features from a DNN. As was already indicated, the output obstacle brought on by understanding different AI algorithms is that when behavioural intelligence data and genetic factors are applied simultaneously, a problem arises (Chen *et al.* 2014, Srivastava *et al.* 2014).

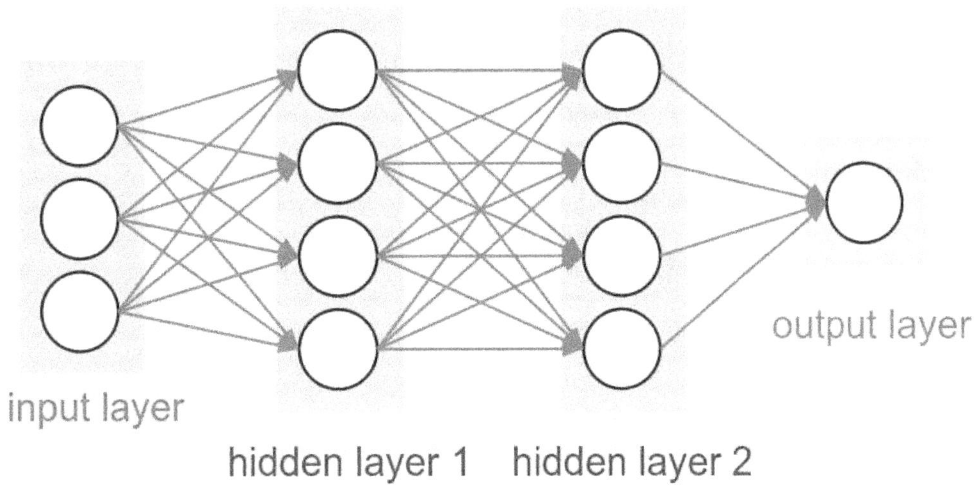

Figure 5.3 Deep Neural Network

An example of a DNN can be seen in Figure 5.3. It consists of layers with weight matrices W and bias vectors b. In order to calculate vector h^1 of the first layer activations of a DNN, we use the following methods:

$$h^{(1)}(x)=\sigma\left(W^{(1)T}x+b^{(1)}\right), \tag{5.4}$$

Assuming $W^{(1)}$ is the weight matrix and $b^{(1)}$ is the bias vector for the first hidden layer, respectively. Using the hidden activations of the preceding layer $h^{(i-1)}$, subsequent hidden layers calculate their hidden activation vector $h^{(i)}$.

$$h^{(i)}(x)=\sigma\left(W^{(i)T}h^{(i-1)}x+b^{(i)}\right) \tag{5.5}$$

Each hidden layer is computed on the basis of a point-wise nonlinearity function $\sigma(z)$. In order to define rectifier nonlinearity, we first define what it is:

$$\sigma(z)=\max(z,0)=\begin{cases} z_i & z_i>0 \\ 0 & z_i\leq 0 \end{cases} \tag{5.6}$$

The output of the DNN's last layer must be a correctly constructed probability distribution across all potential output categories. The *softmax* nonlinearity, which is defined as follows, is used by the DNN's final layer to achieve this.

$$\hat{y}_j = \frac{\exp\left(W^{(L)T}h^{(L-1)}+b^{(L)}\right)}{\sum_{k=1}^{N}\exp\left(W^{(L)T}h^{(L-1)}+b^{(L)}\right)} \tag{5.7}$$

As the output vector, the softmax nonlinearity is used to obtain a well-formed probability distribution over the N output classes. Subsequently, this distribution can be employed in the other loss functions mentioned.

5.4 PROPOSED PSORIASIS DISEASE CLASSIFICATION METHODOLOGY

The proposed approach aims to effectively classify skin images as normal or psoriasis-affected images. Psoriasis is one type of skin disease. Many skin diseases look similar, making it difficult to identify the type of abnormality. To attain this objective a double path cascaded convolution neural network (DPCCNN) is developed. In the cascade CNN, the local and global features of the image are extracted. Three steps, including pre-processing, data augmentation, and classification, make up the suggested methodology. Initially, the skin disease image dataset is collected from the internet. In order to pre-process (noise removal) the images, a median filter is applied. The procedure of data augmentation is executed subsequent to pre-processing. The DPCCNN classifier is then fed the images to determine if each picture is normal or afflicted by psoriasis. The working flow of the presented psoriasis disease classification methodology is given in Figure 5.4.

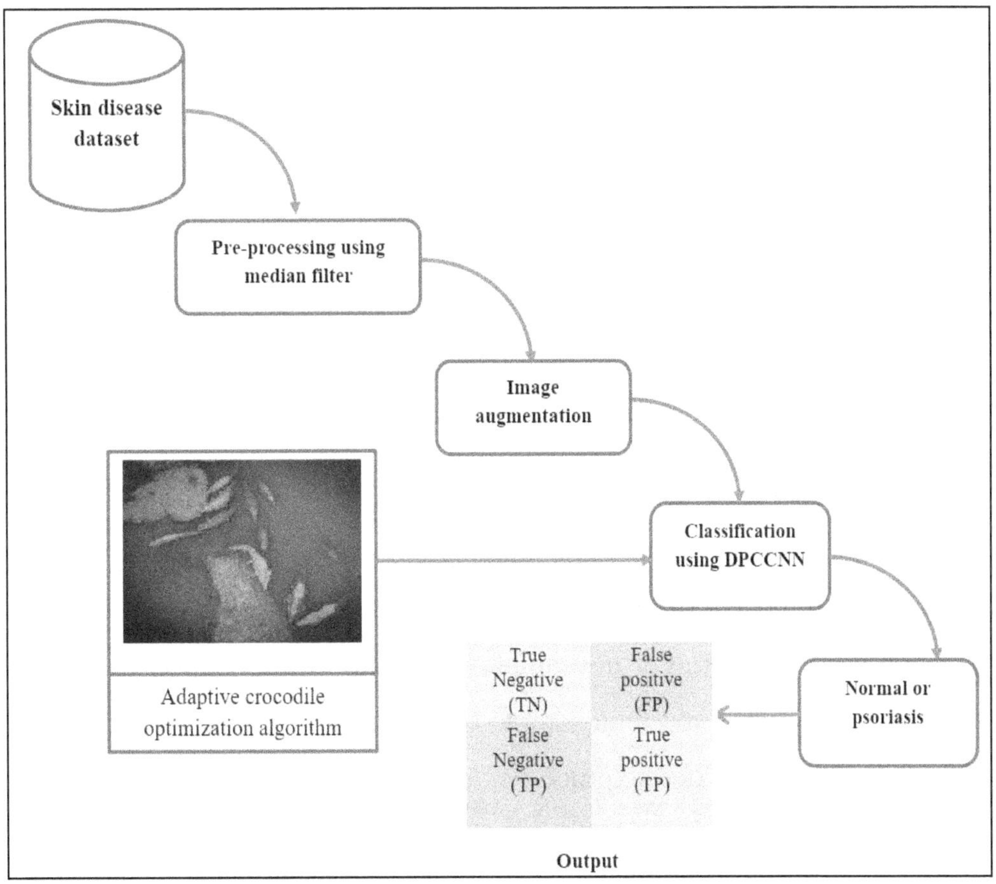

Figure 5.4 Framework for proposed psoriasis disease classification

5.4.1 Noise Removal

Classification involves several steps, including pre-processing. During this phase, the goal is to improve the quality of the input image. To begin with, we gather images from an alternative skin clinic. The collected images are then subjected to a pre-processing step. A median filter is applied as a pre-processing step in this study. Using a median filter, a non-linear digital filtering method, noise in images can be reduced. Consider the skin image, $z_{i,j}$ which has various noises. Each pixel is represented and transformed by the statistical mean of its neighborhood to reduce noise.

5.4.1.1 Median filters

The median filter is the most extensively used OS filter. The methods used to define homomorphic and polynomial filters determine their design and analysis, whilst more heuristic approaches are frequently employed to select order statistic filters. This led to a long period of poorly understood behaviour for the median filter and other similar filters.

Definition of Median Filter

Let the sequences of input and output be represented as {x(i)} and {y(i)}, respectively. Over {x(i)}, a 2N+1 point wide window is slid by a one-dimensional median filter. The middle or median value is utilised as the filter output at each point after the sample within the window has been sorted. In the window centre, the time sample corresponds to the median output. One way to explain the filtering process is as

$$z(i) = \text{median}\,[y(i-N), y(i-(N+1)), \ldots\ldots, y(i), \ldots\ldots, y(i+N)], i \in X \tag{5.8}$$

Running median or moving median are other names for Equation (5.8). The window must append "N" numbers of samples at both the start and finish of the input signal sequence in order for it to reach both the front and back ends. The values of the front end points take the first sample, while the rear end points take the last sample. The following is the definition of the two-dimensional median filtering procedure.

$$z(i,j) = \text{median}\,(y(i+r, j+s)) \qquad (r,s) \in A \text{ and } (i,j) \in X^2 \qquad (5.9)$$

The set $A \subseteq X^2$ defines the neighborhood of the central pixel (i,j). It is called the filter window. The border samples of two dimensional images are processed by replicating them as done in one dimensional median filtering.

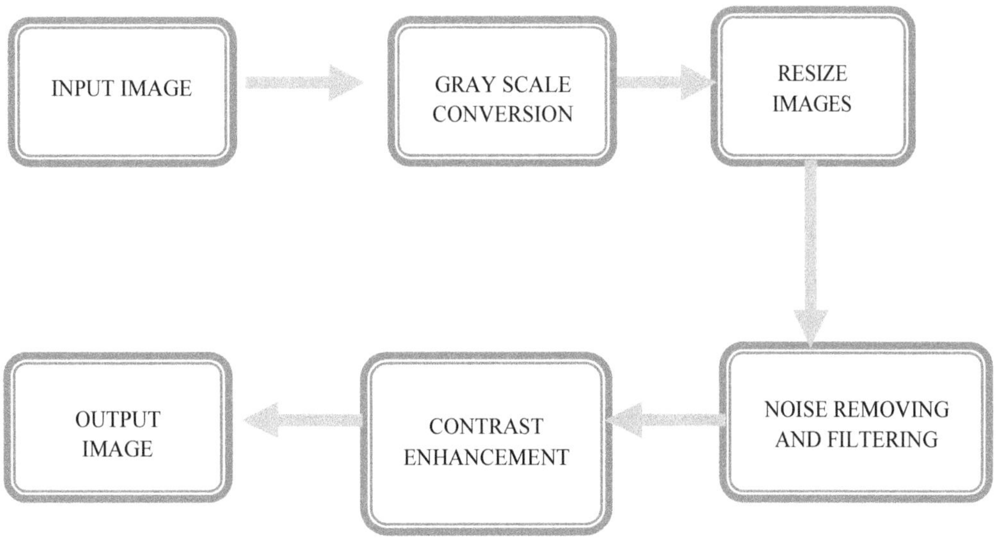

Figure 5.5 Pre-processing using median filters

Edge preservation properties

Edges are essential elements of images that convey important information that is necessary for human visual interpretation. Edge data is essential for image processing and object categorization in addition to its function in perceptual processes. Ataman *et al.* (1981) claim that median filters are excellent in maintaining edges. In particular, these filters effectively suppress noise by functioning as low-pass filters in homogenous regions and adapting to the features of the input. Concurrently, they demonstrate high-pass behaviour in the vicinity of edges, guaranteeing the retention of these crucial characteristics. Images can have edges in any direction (horizontal, vertical, or diagonal), and the median filter's capacity to maintain these edges depends on the filter window's geometry (Nieminen *et al.* 1987; Longbotham & Bovik 1989). While X-shaped filters work best for retaining diagonal edges, cross-shaped windows are best at maintaining horizontal and vertical edges. Square windows work well for maintaining edges in all orientations because they don't have a preferred direction. Since most images have edges pointing in different directions, square-shaped filters are frequently used due to their adaptability.

Statistical properties of median filters

In the L1 sense, the median lowers the following, making it the best location estimator:

$$\sum_{i=1}^{n} |x(i) - T| \rightarrow \min \qquad (5.10)$$

When there is long-tailed noise present, the median filter remains strong. Pitas and Venetsanopoulos (1990) describe the Influence Function (IF), a function that can be used to analyse the impact of an outlier (impulse) on an estimator's performance. Given a distribution F and a sample space X, the estimator T's IF at that distribution is represented as IF (x: T, F). Constants make up the influence function. The median's dependability and robustness are established by these features. Figure 5.6 demonstrates the robustness of the median by showing how the addition of a single outlier, represented by the symbol x(i), has little influence on the median but can have a significant impact on the mean. Furthermore, for distributions with long tails, the asymptotic efficiency of the median is larger than 1.

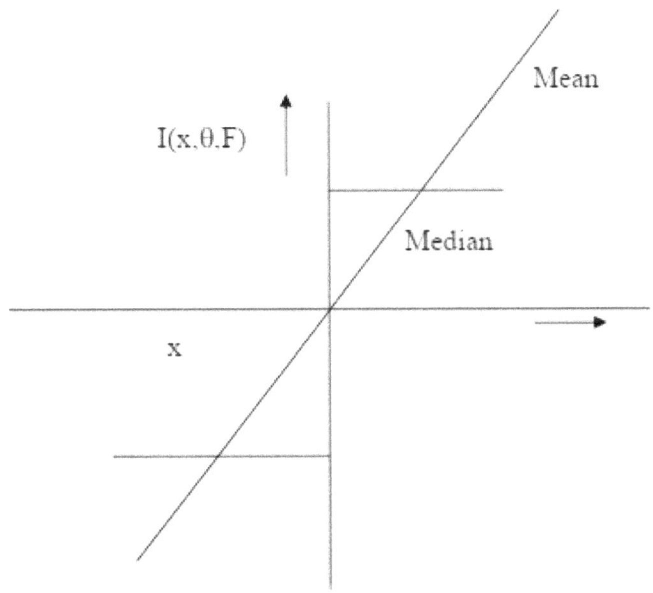

Figure 5.6 Function of influence in relation to an outlier

5.4.2 Image Augmentation

Pre-processing is followed by image augmentation. The dataset's current images can be improved by using image augmentation. In order to improve CNN's performance and generalization, online data augmentation is used to increase the quantity of the training dataset. Images are enlarged by rotating, flipping, cropping, and translating, as well as randomly darkening and brightening them. The images were then scaled down to a fixed size that changed depending on the CNN used.

5.4.3 Proposed Psoriasis Disease Classification using Double Path Cascade

As a result of the pre-processing, the images are directly sent to the CNN classifier to determine whether or not the image is a normal image or one associated with psoriasis. The double path classifier is effective, extracts the local and global features, and combined them to produce the proper output with the help of a FCL.

5.4.4 Double Path Cascade CNN Classifier

This sector has as its primary objective the classification of an image of normal skin or an image depicting psoriasis. A double path cascade CNN classifier is utilized in this paper in order to achieve a better classification output. An image classification technique based on a double-path CNN is proposed in which both local and global features are used. Depending on the size of the kernel, single-path CNNs can target both local and global features. To achieve higher performance, some additional information should be needed. Thus, both local and global image properties are taken into account in this research. Also, further, enhance the classification accuracy, the cascade classifier weight values are optimally selected using the ACO algorithm. The proposed double path cascade CNN classifier structure is given in Figure 5.7.

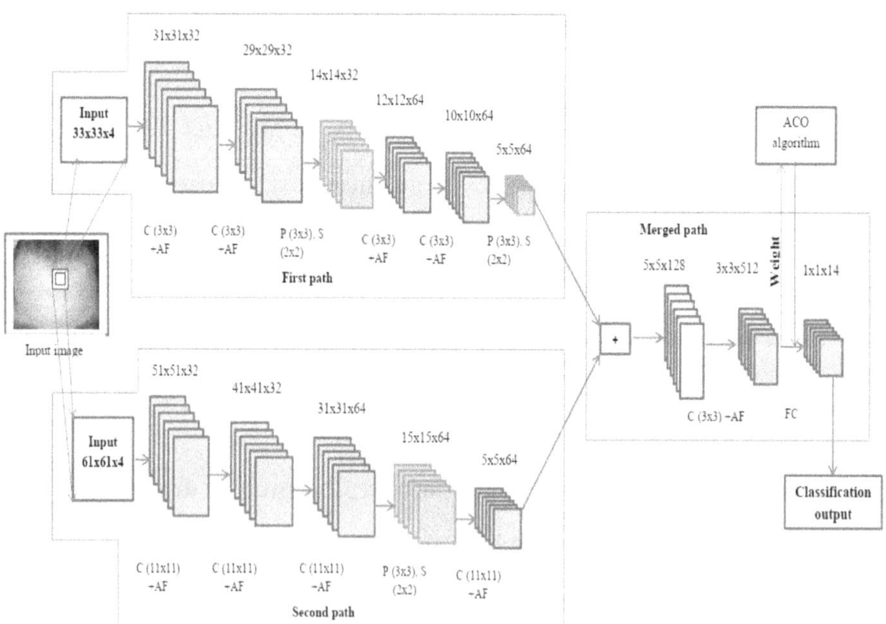

Figure 5.7 Proposed double pathway cascade CNN framework

In this study, we first investigate two separate patches, represented by the letters and, that are both centred on the same pixel in the input retinal image. The system under consideration employs a two-pronged strategy: the first path concentrates on obtaining local characteristics specifically designed for patch processing, while the second path is devoted to obtaining global features from the patches. The number of pooling and convolutional layers in each path varies. Because the deep path (first path) uses small convolutional kernels, more convolutional layers can be stacked with less training weights. On the other hand, the medium-sized kernels (11×11) used in the shallow path (second path) are employed to extract global characteristics from the input patches. Small kernel sizes (3×3) are used in the first path to extract local characteristics from the images. In the end, the feature extraction from both routes is integrated. The output of a convolution layer is sent to the FCL after the feature maps have been created. To determine the optimal weight values for the FCL, the Ant Colony Optimisation (ACO) algorithm is used. The ultimate output is produced by the completely connected layer. Specific details about the features of each layer are given in Table 5.1.

Table 5.1 Parameter details of proposed double path cascade CNN classifier

Layer no	Type of layer	Network input	Size of kernel	stride	Feature map	Activation function	Output
Path 1 (local pathway)							
1	Convolution	33x33x34	3x3	1x1	32	-	31x31x32
2	Activation	31x31x32	-	-	-	ReLU	31x31x32
3	Convolution	31x31x32	3x3	1x1	32	-	29x29x32
4	Activation	29x29x32	-	-	-	ReLU	29x29x32
5	Max-pooling	29x29x32	3x3	2x2	-	-	14x14x32
6	Convolution	14x14x32	3x3	1x1	64	-	12x12x64
7	Activation	12x12x64	-	-	-	ReLU	12x12x128
8	Convolution	12x12x128	3x3	1x1	64	-	10x10x64
9	Activation	10x10x64	-	-	-	ReLU	10x10x64
10	Max-pooling	10x10x64	2x2	2x2	-	-	5x5x64

Table 5.1 (Continued)

Layer no	Type of layer	Network input	Size of kernel	stride	Feature map	Activation function	Output
Path 2(Global pathway)							
1	Convolution	61x61x4	11x11	1x1	32		51x51x32
2	Activation	51x51x32	-	-	-	ReLU	51x51x32
3	Convolution	51x51x32	11x11	1x1	32		41x41x32
4	Activation	41x41x32	-	-	-	ReLU	41x41x32
5	Convolution	41x41x32	11x11	1x1	64		31x31x64
6	Activation	31x31x64	-	-	-	ReLU	31x31x64
7	Max-Pooling	31x31x64	3x3	2x2	-		15x15x64
8	Convolution	15x15x64	11x11	1x1	64		5x5x64
9	Activation	5x5x64	-	-	-	ReLU	5x5x64
Merged path (global pathway +Local pathway)							
1	Convolution	5x5x(64+64)	3x3	1x1	512		3x3x512
2	Activation	3x3x512	-	-	-	ReLU	3x3x512
3	Fully connected	3x3x512	3x3	1x1	4		1x1x14
4	Activation	1x1x14	-	-	-	ReLU	1x1x14

The loss of classification in this study is measured using the softmax log loss function. As per Muhaba *et al.* (2022), the forward transform of softmax log loss can be expressed as follows:

$$Z = -\log \frac{e^{x_1}}{\sum_{j=1}^{n} e^{x_j}} = \log\left(\sum_{j=1}^{n} e^{x_j}\right) - x_i = \log(S) - x_i \tag{5.11}$$

$$S = \sum_{i=1}^{n} e^{x_i} \tag{5.12}$$

where i denote the class index and n denote the number of classes. During the back propagation, $\frac{\partial z}{\partial x}$ is calculated by equation (5.1).

$$\frac{\partial z}{\partial x} = -\frac{1}{p_i}\left(\left[\delta_{ij} p_i\right] - p p_i^T\right) = -\frac{1}{p_i}\left([0,\ldots,p_i,\ldots,0] - p\,[p_1,\ldots,p_c]\right) - [0,\ldots,1_i,\ldots,0] \tag{5.13}$$

5.4.5 Weight Optimization using ACO Algorithm

The ACO algorithm is used in this part to pick the weight values in the cascade CNN in the best possible way. This programme mimics the hunting technique of crocodiles and is based on their behaviour. This population-based technique can be used to optimisation challenges using swarm intelligence. The author separates the crocodiles into two groups—chasers and ambushers—during the hunting procedure. Chasing crocodiles are larger than other crocodiles, and instead of catching fish, they chase fish toward the shore with their powerful tail. Smaller ambushers wait in the shallows and try to pick on the fish.

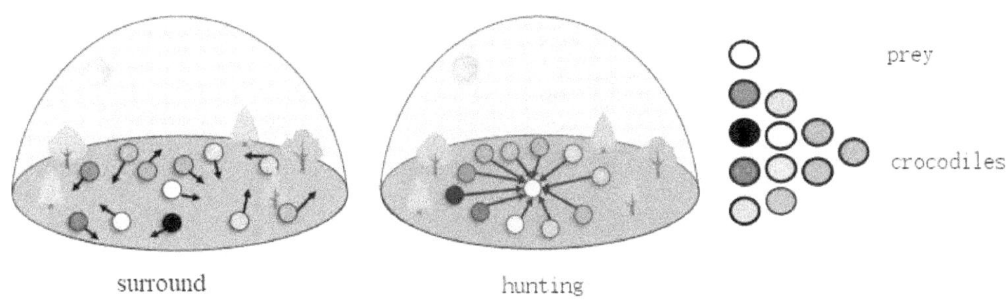

Figure 5.8 ACO algorithm

To enhance the updation function Levy flight strategy is adapted with the crocodile optimization algorithm. The following describes the weight optimisation procedure sequentially:

Step 1: Solution initialization: Solution initiation is a vital phase for all optimization problems.. In this section, the FCLs' weight values are optimally selected. So, the solution includes weight values. The solution is represented as a crocodile. In ACO, initially, the solutions are initialized randomly. These random solutions form the initial population of crocodiles. The initial solution format is given in Equation (5.14).

$$P = \{A_i\} \ , i \leq 1 \leq n \tag{5.14}$$

$$A_1 = [w_{11} \ \ w_{12} \ \ w_{1n}] \tag{5.15}$$

where, P represent the population, A_i represent the solutions and w_i represent the weight value. In this stage, we also initialize the number of populations, maximum number of iterations and other parameters present in the CSO algorithm.

Step 2: Objective function calculation: The Objective function of each solution is determined after the solutions are initiated. Objective function are considered to be the most accurate functions. In order to evaluate Objective function , the following equations are used;

$$Fitness = Maximum(Accuracy) \tag{5.16}$$

$$P = \{A_i\} \ , i \leq 1 \leq n \tag{5.17}$$

Step 3: Chasing the prey: In this step, the chaser's behavior is stimulated. Because chasers are nearer to prey, the first 50% of crocodiles (solutions) are grouped to create chasers. Consequently, the other 50 % of the solutions consist of ambushers. Compared to the chaser group, the ambusher's group has more distance from the prey. As a result, the distance between the prey and the crocodiles determines the order in which the solutions are found. In contrast to ambushers, chasers have greater distance values from their target. As indicated earlier, chasers do not capture the prey but chase the prey to the shore and shallows. The behavior of chasing prey is given in Equations (5.18) and (5.19).

$$d = \left| x^{t}_{prey} - x^{i,t}_{chaser} \right| \ \forall i \tag{5.18}$$

$$\begin{cases} x^{i,t+1}_{chaser} = \left(x^{i,t}_{chaser} - \beta\, r.d\right) \times Levy(\gamma) & \forall i\ d < \alpha \\ x^{i,t+1}_{chaser} = \left(\bar{x}_{rand} - \beta \bar{r}.d\right) \times Levy(\gamma) & \forall i\ d \geq \alpha \end{cases} \tag{5.19}$$

Where;

x^{t}_{prey} → Prey position at iteration t

$x^{i,t}_{chaser}$ →Position of the crocodile i^{th} at iteration t

$\bar{x}_{rand}$ → Random vector position

β →Uniform distribution with a 0–3 range of variation

r → Random value generated between 0-1.

d → Distance between the ith chaser and the prey.

$Levy(\gamma)$ → Levy flight strategy

$$Levy(\gamma) \sim u = t^{-1-\gamma}, \quad 0 < \gamma \leq 2 \tag{5.20}$$

The levy flight step length can be evaluated using Equation (5.21)

$$s = \frac{U}{|V|^{1/\gamma}} \tag{5.21}$$

where, U and V represent the Gaussian distribution which is calculated using equation (5.22).

$$U \sim N\left(0, \sigma^2_U\right),\ V \sim N\left(0, \sigma^2_V\right) \tag{5.22}$$

$$\sigma_U = \left(\frac{\Gamma(1+\beta).\sin\left(\pi\beta/2\right)}{\Gamma\left((1+\beta)/2\right).\beta.2^{(\beta-1)/2}} \right)^{1/\beta} \tag{5.23}$$

$$\sigma_V = 1 \tag{5.24}$$

Each chaser in the first group moved toward the prey with a positive coefficient using (5.19) if $d < \alpha$. Besides, random search is done if $d \geq \alpha$. Briefly say that the attack is done by chasers if the chasers are close to the prey. Else, by a random approach close to the prey.

Step 4: Attacking to prey: Here, the ambushers capture their target at the very final level. Followers attempt to lead the victim to the final location or domain of the ambusher. The attackers are presumed to update their location using Equations (5.25), (5.26), and (5.27) in order to replicate the attack phase.

$$d = \left| x^{t}_{prey} - x^{i,t}_{ambusher} \right| \quad \forall i \tag{5.25}$$

$$A = \frac{apc + apa + prey\ position}{3} \tag{5.26}$$

$$\begin{cases} x^{i,t+1}_{ambusher} = \left(d.\cos(2\pi) + x^{t}_{i,prey}\right) \times Levy(\gamma) & \forall i\ d < \alpha \\ x^{i,t+1}_{ambusher} = \left(x^{i,t}_{a} - \beta\left(A - x_{a}\right)\right) \times Levy(\gamma) & \forall i\ d \geq \alpha \end{cases} \tag{5.27}$$

where;

$x^{i,t}_{a}$ → Position of ith ambusher at iteration t

d → Distance between the ambushers and the prey

apc → Chasers Average position

apa → Ambusher's Average position

Each ambusher swims around the prey with a rotational motion using (5.27) if $d < \alpha$. Depend on the average of the position of the all group of chasers, ambushers, and the prey, the position of ambushers is updated using (5.27) if $d \geq \alpha$.

Step 5: Termination criteria: All of these stages are carried out until the ideal weight or solution is obtained. The algorithm will stop working otherwise. The procedure of classification is given the chosen ideal weight value.

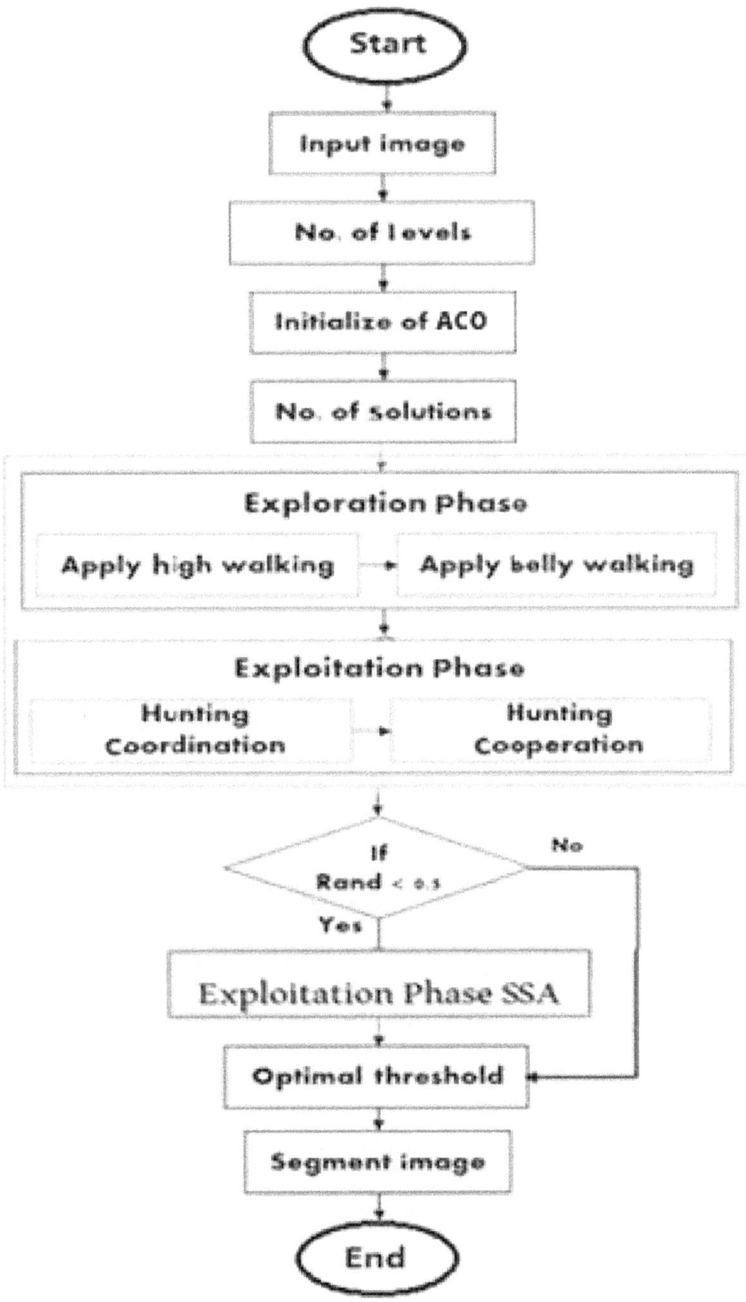

Figure 5.9 Adaptive crocodile optimisation (ACO) method

Algorithm 5.1: Weight optimization using ACO algorithm

Input: Weight parameters of CNN

Output: Optimal weight parameters

1. Initialize the solutions.

2. Evaluate the fitness for each solution using (5.16)

Chasing the prey

3. Calculate distance between the chaser and the prey using (5.18).

4. **If** $d < \alpha$

5. The chaser in the first group used (5.19) to move with a positive coefficient in the direction of the prey.

6. Else

7. Random search is done using (5.19).

8. **End If**

Attacking to prey

9. Calculate distance between the chaser and the prey using (5.25).

10. Calculate average position of all group using (5.26).

11. **If** $d < \alpha$

12. Each ambusher uses a circular motion to swim around the target (5.27).

13. **Else**

The position of ambushers is updated using (5.27).

14. **End If**

15. Continue the algorithm until finding the solution, else terminate the algorithm.

5.5 RESULTS AND DISCUSSION

An experimental study based on the proposed approach is presented in this section. The recommended method for psoriasis disease diagnosis is simulated using Matlab version 2020a on a Windows 10 OS, Intel core i3 CPU, and 4GB RAM machine. The efficacy of the suggested methodology is evaluated by a variety of metrics, including recall, F-measure, NPV, MCC, TPR, FPR, and FNR. Psoriasis images from private clinics are gathered for this study. The following is a list of example images used in the experiment;

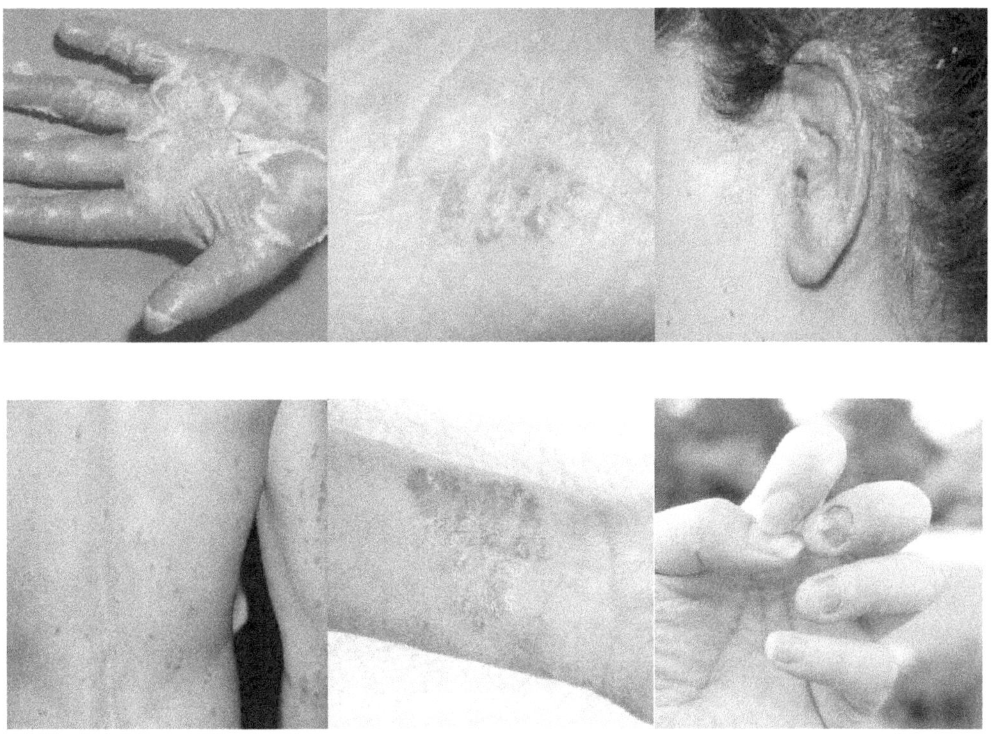

Figure 5.10 Sample images used in the experiment

5.6 EXPERIMENTAL RESULTS

Using various criteria, the classification performance using the DPCCNN approach is examined. Additionally, the effectiveness of the Deep Neural Network (DNN), Conventional CNN, and Single Path Cascade CNN (SPCCNN) classification algorithms is contrasted with that of the DPCCNN. We concluded from this discussion that the suggested DPCCNN-based categorization model outperforms SPCCNN, CNN, and DNN in terms of real results. For the following reasons: i) the SPCCNN model only took into account local variables for classification; ii) CNN's FCLs make training less time-consuming due to insufficient weight distribution or connection iii) The DNN gives each attribute the same weight, which may have an impact on classification accuracy.

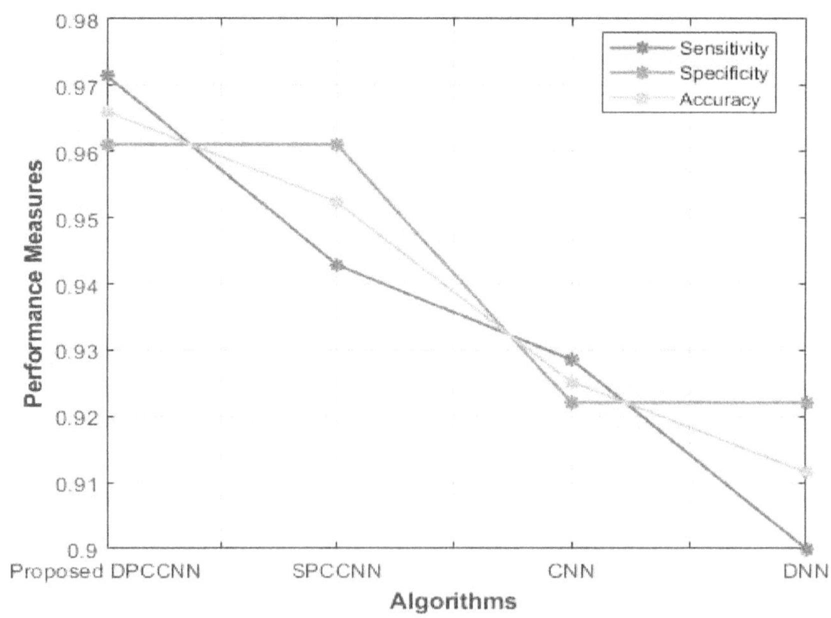

Figure 5.11 Analyzing the accuracy, sensitivity, and specificity of different classification algorithms

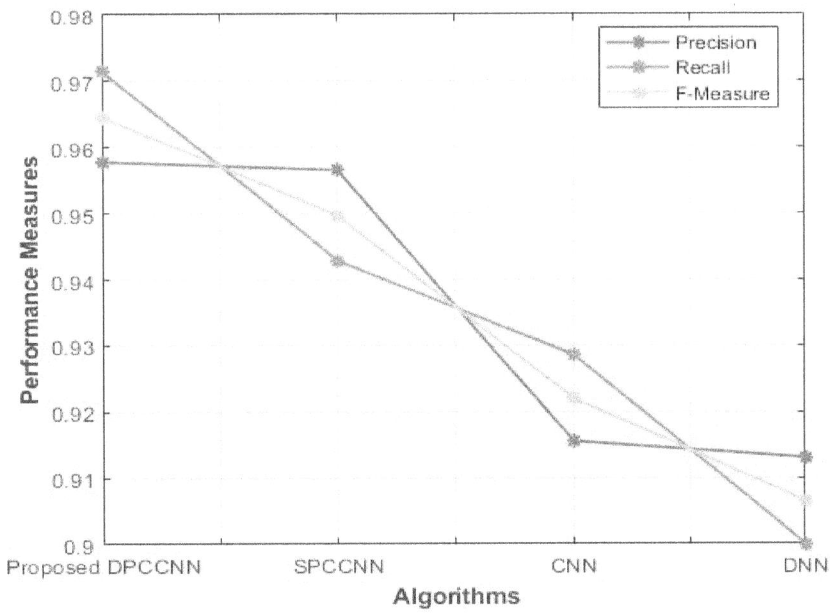

Figure 5.12 The evaluation of several classification techniques comparisons using Precision, F-Measure and Recall

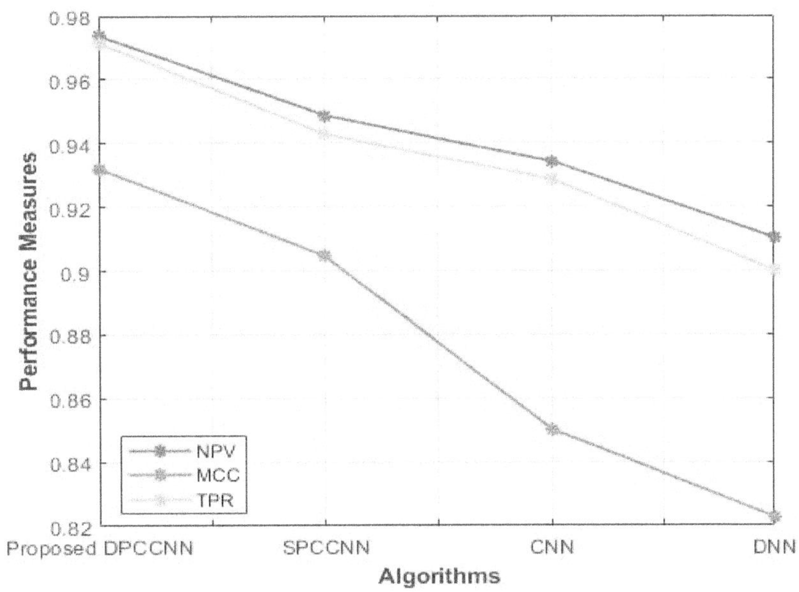

Figure 5.13 NPV, MCC, and TPR analyses of various classification algorithms

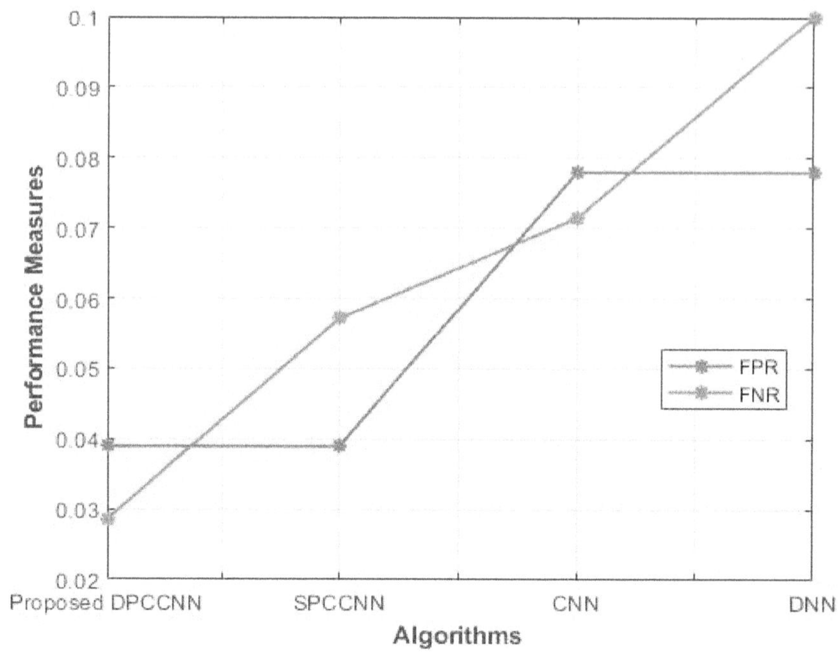

Figure 5.14 Comparative evaluation of different classification methods using FPR and FNR

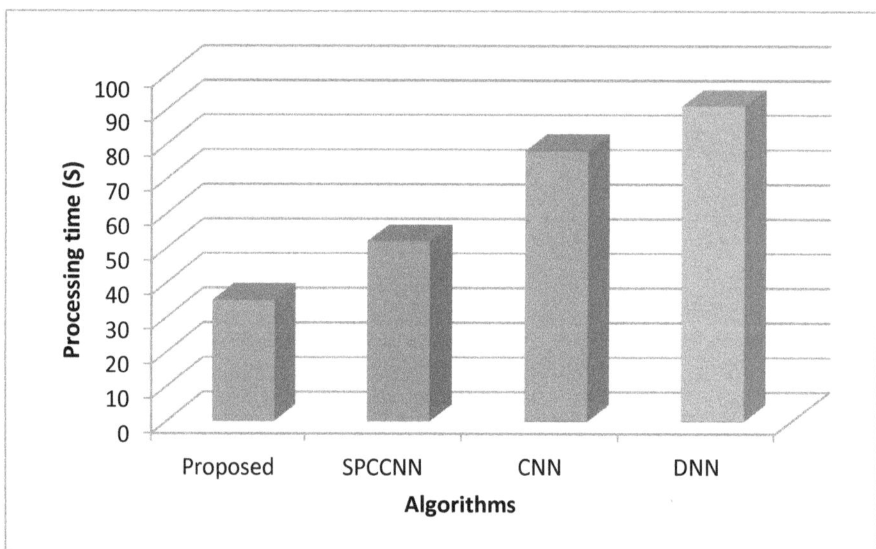

Figure 5.15 Processing time of different classification methods

Figure 5.11 illustrates a comparison of the specificity, sensitivity, and accuracy of several classification algorithms. When compared with DNN and CNN-based categorization, SPCCNN achieved the highest accuracy of 94.2%. However, this research improves the classification performance of

SPCCNN by introducing a secondary route to extract the global features of images and optimising its weight parameters with ACOA. As a result, the suggested DPCCNN achieved 96.59% accuracy. Additionally, the ACO algorithm-based weight optimisation and local and global characteristics were responsible for the highest levels of sensitivity and specificity of 97.1% and 96.1%, respectively. Figure 5.12 presents the results of comparison analysis based on F-measure, recall, and precision metrics. By analyzing Figure 5.12, the proposed model achieved a high degree of precision of 96.7%. This compares to 94.6% for SPCCNN-based classification, 91.5% for CNN-based classification, and 91.3% for DNN-based classification. Comparing the suggested method to the current classifiers, it achieved a high maximum recall and F-measure of 97.14% and 96.45%, respectively. In figure 5.13, we analyse the performance of the proposed strategy using NPV, MCC, and TPR. Compared to other approaches that are now in use, including SPCCNN, CNN, and DNN, which represent 0.9487, 0.9342, and 0.9102, respectively, it demonstrates a higher NPV of 0.9736. Comparably, we achieved a higher MCC of 0.93, which is comparable to 0.90 for training with DNNs, 0.85 for CNNs, and 0.90 for SPCCNNs-based classification. In addition, we achieved the highest TPR of 0.97 in comparison to alternative approaches. Figure 5.14 shows the performance evaluation of the false positive and false negative rates for the suggested method. Among the current techniques, including SPCCNN, CNN, and DNN, which represent 0.0571, 0.071, and 0.1, respectively, it displays a low FNR of 0.028. In addition, our strategy achieved the lowest FPR in contrast to an alternative. It is evident from the results section that, in comparison to other classifiers, the planned model produced the best results. The weights were optimised because of the dual path cascade CNN and ACO algorithm. Figure 5.15 depicts the processing time of different classification methods. As depicted in the graph, processing time of the proposed scheme is reduced to 33%, 55% and 62% than that of SPCCNN, CNN, and DNN respectively.

5.7 EXISTING WORK COMPARED WITH THE PROPOSED METHOD

They took into account the form, colour, and GLCM texture feature areas. Table 5.2 displays the comparing findings based on accuracy. In this work, we utilized DPCCNN classifier for the classification process. For comparison, in this paper, we utilize five works. Dynamic graph cutting and naïve Bayes classifier were used by Balaji *et al.* (2021) to classify skin diseases. Wei *et al.* (2018), they consider the GLCM texture features and color features for skin disease prediction. ANN-based skin disease classification is presented in (Bajaj *et al.* 2018). They consider the different sets of features for classification. Patnaik *et al.* (2018), the author discussed the CNN-based skin disease classification. Similarly, in Macatangay*et al.* (2016), KNN-based classification was discussed. They took into account the form, colour, and GLCM texture feature areas. Table 5.2 displays the comparing findings based on accuracy.

Table 5.2 Comparison results of proposed and state-of-the-art works

Research work	Accuracy	Sensitivity	Specificity
dynamic graph cut and Naïve Bayes classifier (Balaji *et al.* 2020)	72.7	71.25	74.79
SVM (Wei *et al.* 2018)	90	-	-
ANN (Bajaj *et al.* 2018)	90	-	-
CNN (Patnaik *et al.*2018)	88	-	-
Ensemble (Macatangay *et al.* 2017)	65.63	-	-
Proposed	96.59	97	96

As illustrated in Table 5.2, the planned model achieved an improved classification accuracy of 96.59% which is 65.63% for (Macatangay *et al.* 2017), 88% for (Patnaik *et al.* 2018), 90% for (Wei *et al.* 2018, Bajaj *et al.* 2018), and 72.7% for (Balaji *et al.* 2020). From the results section, we clearly understand, the planned model attained higher accuracy compared to existing research work. This is due to automatic global and local feature extraction, weight optimization using the ACO algorithm, and double-path CNN. Psoriasis disease can be easily identified using this method. Early detection is reducing severe infection and spreads in the human body. Therefore, this method is recommended for medicine. The obtained results will help the patient to go further treatment.

5.8 SUMMARY

This research offered a technique for categorising cutaneous psoriasis. A unique classifier, DPCCNN, has been created to fulfil this goal. The suggested method extracted both local and global characteristics individually. To improve classification performance, the ACO algorithm is used to choose the weight optimum. The double route cascade CNN improves classification performance over the existing single path cascade CNN, conventional CNN, and DNN classifier. A range of indicators were employed to assess the success of the suggested strategy. The given method achieved a maximum accuracy of 96.7%. In the future, we will concentrate on many sorts of psoriasis skin problems.

CHAPTER 6

CONCLUSION AND FUTURE WORK

6.1 CONCLUSION

In this study, an AChOA-CNN-based segmentation method was introduced to improve the accuracy of segmenting images of skin affected by psoriasis. It was necessary to normalize and scale the input images of psoriasis during the preprocessing step. AChOA is used to adjust the weight and bias settings of the convolutional layer once the optimized CNN receives the preprocessed images. A chaotic sequence taken from a tent map has been used to enhance the search abilities of the ChOA algorithm. The segmented images were eliminated of artefacts using the threshold module. Segmentation models based on CNN, SVM, ANN, and RF have been compared to see how well they work with the segmentation model that is offered. The article's findings demonstrate that the proposed segmentation model, which is based on AChOA-CNN, obtained 97% accuracy, 90% JI, and 96% DC.

In second phase, a classification scheme for skin psoriasis was proposed. An innovative classifier called DPCCNN has been created to accomplish this goal. The local and global characteristics were retrieved independently using the suggested methodology. The ACO algorithm is introduced to choose the weight optimum in order to enhance classification performance. Over the single path cascade CNN, conventional CNN, and DNN classifiers currently in use, the double path cascade CNN improves classification performance. A range of indicators have been employed to assess the effectiveness of the suggested strategy. The greatest accuracy of the proposed method was 96.7%. We will concentrate on various skin psoriasis conditions in the future.

6.2 FUTURE SCOPE

- Future applications of the proposed techniques will be made on backdrops with a wider range of complexity.
- It is anticipated that hybrid deep learning algorithms will be developed in the future in order to enhance the performance of the disease detection model.
- More work needs to be done in identifying numerous psoriatic lesions in full-body images of psoriasis patients.
- The creation of any hybrid optimisations to improve performance will be the future of psoriasis classification.
- In the future, we aim to use more sophisticated neural networks to test the usefulness of the proposed data augmentation approach on datasets with additional modulation schemes.

REFERENCES

1. Aijaz, SF, Khan, SJ, Azim, F, Shakeel, CS & Hassan, U β0ββ, ‗Deep learning application for effective classification of different types of psoriasis', Journal of Healthcare Engineering,vol.2022, Article ID 7541583, p. 12.

2. Al-Masni, MA, Kim, DH & Kim, TS β0β0, ‗Multiple skin lesions diagnostics via integrated deep convolutional networks for segmentation and classification', Computer Methods and Programs in Biomedicine, vol. 190, p.105351.

3. Al-Saffar, AA, Tao, H & Talab, MA β017, ‗Review of deep convolution neural network in image classification', International Conference on Radar, Antenna, Microwave, Electronics, and Telecommunications (ICRAMET), pp. 26-31. IEEE.

4. Amit, Y & Geman, D 1997, ‗Shape quantization and recognition with randomized trees', Neural Computation, vol. 9, no. 7, pp. 1545-1588.

5. Armstrong, AW, Gelfand, JM & Garg A β01γ, ‗Outcomes research in psoriasisand psoriatic arthritis using large databases and research networks: areport from the GRAPPA Annual Meeting', Journal of Rheumatol, vol. 41, no. 6, pp. 1233–1236.

6. Arora, R, Raman, B, Nayyar, K & Awasthi, R β0β1, ‗Automated skin lesion segmentation using attention-based deep convolutional neural network. Biomedical Signal Processing and Control, vol. 65, p.102358.

7. Arora, R, Raman, B, Nayyar, K & Awasthi, R β0β1, ‗Automated skin lesion segmentation using attention-based deep convolutional neural network', Biomedical Signal Processing and Control, vol. 65, p. 102358.

8. Arunkumar, TR & Jayanna, HS β0ββ, ‗A Novel Light-Weight Approach for the Classification of Different Types of Psoriasis Disease Using Depth Wise Separable Convolution Neural Networks', Indian Journal of Science and Technology, vol. 15, no. 13, pp.561-569.

9. Bajaj, L, Kumar, H & Hasija, Y β018, _Automated System for Prediction of Skin Disease using Image Processing and Machine Learning', International Journal of Computer Applications, vol. 180, no. 19, pp. 9–12.

10. Bajwa, MN, Muta, K, Malik, MI, Siddiqui, SA, Braun, SA, Homey, B, Dengel, A & Ahmed, S β0β0, _Computer-aided diagnosis of skin diseases using deep neural networks', Applied Sciences, vol. 10, no. 7, p. 2488.

11. Balaji, VR, Suganthi, ST, Rajadevi, R, Kumar, VK, Balaji, BS & Pandiyan, S β0β0, _Skin disease detection and segmentation using dynamic graph cut algorithm and classification through Naive Bayes classifier', Measurement, vol. 163, p.107922.

12. Balaji, VR, Suganthi, ST, Rajadevi, R, Kumar, VK, Balaji, BS & Pandiyan, S β0β0, _Skin disease detection and segmentation using dynamic graph cut algorithm and classification through Naive Bayes Classifier', Measurement, vol. 16γ, p. 1079ββ.

13. Birkenfeld, JS, Tucker-Schwartz, JM, Soenksen, LR, Avilés-Izquierdo, JA & Marti-Fuster, B β0β0, _Computer-aided classification of suspicious pigmented lesions using wide-field images', Computer Methods and Programs in Biomedicine, vol. 195, p.105631.

14. Breiman, L β001, _Bagging Predictors', Machine Learning, vol. 24, no. 2, pp. 123–140.

15. Breiman, L β001, _Random Forests', Machine Learning, vol. 45, no. 1, pp. 5–32.

16. Burges, C 1998, _A tutorial on support vector machines for pattern recognition', In ―Data Mining and Knowledge Discovery‖. Kluwer Academic Publishers, Boston, vol. 2.

17. Cameron, JB & Voohees, S β014, _History of Psoriasis', London: Springer.

18. Chatterjee, S, Dey, D & Munshi, S β019, _Integration of morphological preprocessing and fractal based feature extraction with recursive feature elimination for skin lesion types classification', Computer Methods and Programs in Biomedicine, vol. 178, pp.201-218.

19. Chatterjee, S, Dey, D, Munshi, S & Gorai, S β019, _Extraction of features from cross correlation in space and frequency domains for classification of skin lesions', Biomedical Signal Processing and Control, vol. 53, p.101581.

20. Chen, W, Chen, S, Zhang, H & Wu, T β017, _A hybrid prediction model for type 2 diabetes using K-means and decision tree', 8th IEEE International Conference on Software Engineering and Service Science (ICSESS), China, pp.386-390.

21. Chen, Y, Lin, Z, Zhao, X, Wang, G & Gu, Y β014, _Deep learning based classification of hyperspectral data', IEEE Journal of Selected Topics in Applied Earth Observations and Remote Sensing, vol. 7, no. 6, pp. 2094–2107.

22. Chirstianini, N & Shawe Taylor, J β000, _An Introduction to Support Vector Machine', Cambridge University, University Press.

23. Coondoo, A β01β, _The role of cytokines in the patho-mechanism of cutaneous disorders', Indian Journal dermatology, vol. 57, pp. 90-96.

24. Cortes, C & Vapnik, V 1995, _Support vector networks', Machine Learning, vol. 20, pp. 273–297.

25. Dash, M, Londhe, N, Ghosh, S, Raj, R & Sonawane, R β0β0 _A cascaded deep convolution neural network based CADx system for psoriasis lesion segmentation and severity assessment', Applied Soft Computing, vol. 91, p. 106240.

26. Dash, M, Londhe, N, Ghosh, S, Semwal, A & Sonawane, R 2019, _PsLSNet: Automated psoriasis skin lesion segmentation using modified U-Net-based fully convolutional network', Biomedical Signal Processing and Control, vol. 52, pp. 226-237.

27. Dash, M, Londhe, ND, Ghosh, S, Raj, R & Sonawane, RS β0β0, _A cascaded deep convolution neural network based CADx system for psoriasis lesion segmentation and severity assessment', Applied Soft Computing, vol. 91, p.106240.

28. Dash, M, Londhe, ND, Ghosh, S, Semwal, A & Sonawane, RS 2019, _PsLSNet: Automated psoriasis s kin lesion segmentation using modified U-Net-based fully convolutional network', Biomedical Signal Processing and Control, vol. 52, pp. 226-237.

29. Dash, M, Londhe, ND, Ghosh, S, Shrivastava, VK & Sonawane, RS β0β0, ‗Swarm intelligence based clustering technique for automated lesion detection and diagnosis of psoriasis', Computational Biology and Chemistry, vol. 86, p.107247.

30. de Korte, J, Sprangers, MA, Mombers, FM & Bos, JD β004, ‗Quality of life in patients with psoriasis: a systematic literature review', Journal of Investigative Dermatology Symposium Proceedings, vol. 9, no. 2, pp. 140-147.

31. Dietterich, TG β000, ‗An experimental comparison of three methods for constructing ensembles of decision trees', Mach Learn, vol. 40, pp. 139–157.

32. Divya, G, Rajitha, P, Swati Gupta, Jayakumar, R & Sabitha, M 2016, ‗Acitretin and aloeemodin loaded chitin nanogel for the treatment of psoriasis', European Journal of Pharmaceutics and Biopharmaceutics, vol. 107, pp. 97-109.

33. Duda R & Hart, P 197γ, ‗Pattern Classification and Scene Analysis', Wiley, New York.

34. El-Darouti, M & Hay, RA β010, ‗Psoriasis: Highlights on pathogenesis, adjuvant therapy and treatment of resistant and problematic cases', Journal of Egyptian Women Dermatologic Society, vol. 7, no. 1, pp. 64-70.

35. Ge, Z, Demyanov, S, Chakravorty, R, Bowling, A & Garnavi, R 2017, ‗Skin disease recognition using deep saliency features and multimodal learning of dermoscopy and clinical images', In Medical Image Computing and Computer Assisted Intervention–MICCAI: β0th International Conference, Quebec City, QC, Canada, September 11-13, Proceedings, Springer International Publishing, vol. 3, no. 20, pp. 250-258.

36. Gelfand, JM & Yeung, H β01β, ‗Metabolic syndrome in patients with psoriaticdisease', Journal of Rheumatology Supplement, vol. 89, pp. 24–28.

37. George, Y, Aldeen, M & Garnavi, R β017, ‗A pixel-based skin segmentation in psoriasis images using committee of machine learning classifiers', International Conference on Digital Image Computing: Techniques and Applications (DICTA), pp. 1-8. IEEE.

38. George, Y, Aldeen, M & Garnavi, R β017, _Automatic psoriasis lesion segmentation in two-dimensional skin images using multiscale superpixel clustering', Journal of Medical Imaging, vol. 4, no. 4, pp. 044004-044004.

39. George, Y, Aldeen, M & Garnavi, R β018, _Psoriasis image representation using patch-based dictionary learning for erythema severity scoring', Computerized Medical Imaging and Graphics, vol. 66, pp. 44-55.

40. George, Y, Aldeen, M & Garnavi, R β019, _Automatic scale severity assessment method in psoriasis skin images using local descriptors', IEEE Journal of Biomedical and Health Informatics, vol. 24, no. 2, pp.577-585.

41. George, Yasmeen M, Mohammad Aldeen & Rahil Garnavi 2017, _Automatic psoriasis lesion segmentation in two-dimensional skin images using multiscale superpixel clustering', Journal of Medical Imaging, vol. 4, no. 4, p. 044004.

42. George, Yasmeen, Mohammad Aldeen & Rahil Garnavi β016, _Pixel-based skin segmentation in psoriasis images', γ8th Annual International Conference of the IEEE Engineering in Medicine and Biology Society (EMBC), IEEE, pp. 1352-1356.

43. Godin, B & Touitou, E β007, _Transdermal skin delivery: Predictions for humans from in vivo, ex vivo and animal models', Advanced drug delivery reviews, vol. 59, pp. 1152-1161.

44. Griffiths, CE & Barker, JN β007, _Pathogenesis and clinical features of psoriasis',Lancet, vol. 370, no. 9583, pp. 263-271.

45. Griffiths, CEM, Christophers, E, Barker, JNWN, Chalmers, RJG, Chimenti, S, Krueger, GG, Leonardi, C, Menter, A, Ortonne, JP & Fry, L β007, _A classification of psoriasis vulgaris according to phenotype', British Journal of Dermatology, vol. 156, no. 2, pp. 258-262.

46. Gu, Z, Cheng, J, Fu, H, Zhou, K, Hao, H, Zhao, Y, Zhang, T, Gao, S & Liu, J 2019, _Ce-net: Context encoder network for 2d medical image segmentation', IEEE Transactions on Medical Imaging, vol. 38, no. 10, pp. 2281-2292.

47. Himani Bhavsar & Mahesh H Panchal β01β, _A review on Support Vector Machine for Data Classification', Intl. Journal of Advanced Research in Computer Engineering and Technology, vol.1, no.10.

48. Hrehorow, E, Salomon, J, Matusiak, L, Reich, A & Szepietowski, JC β01β, _Patients with psoriasis feel stigmatized‘, Acta Derm Venereol, vol. 92, no. 1, pp. 67-72.

49. Hussain, S, Anwar, SM & Majid, M β017, _Brain tumor segmentation using cascaded deep convolutional neural network‘, γ9th Annual International Conference of the IEEE Engineering in Medicine and Biology Society (EMBC). IEEE, pp. 1998-2001.

50. Isa, NM, Amir, A, Ilyas, MZ, Razalli, MS β019, _Motor imagery classification in Brain computer interface (BCI) based on EEG signal by using machine learning technique‘, Bulletin of Electrical Engineering and Informatics, vol. 8, no. 1, pp. 269-75.

51. Jadali, Z, Izad, M, Eslami, MB, Mansouri, P, Safari, R, Bayatian, P, Mirshafiey, A & Salehi Nodeh, AR β007, _Th1/Thβ cytokines in psoriasis‘, Iran J Publ Health, vol. 36, pp. 87-91.

52. Jampani, V, Gadde, R & Gehler, PV β015, _Efficient facade segmentation using auto-context‘, In: Proceedings: IEEE-winter conference on applications of computer vision, WACV‘15, pp. 10γ8–1045

53. Joshi, A & Gautam, P β0β0, _An Implementation of Hybrid method towards the Privacy of HealthCare Record‘, In 2nd International Conference on Data, Engineering and Applications (IDEA), pp. 1-5. IEEE.

54. Khatibi, T, Rezaei, N, Ataei Fashtami, L & Totonchi, M 2021, _Proposing a novel unsupervised stack ensemble of deep and conventional image segmentation (SEDCIS) method for localizing vitiligo lesions in skin images‘, Skin Research and Technology, vol. 27, no. 2, pp. 126-137.

55. Khishe Mohammad & Mohammad Reza Mosavi β0β0, _Chimp optimization algorithm‘, Expert Systems with Applications, vol. 149, p. 113338.

56. Kim, KB & Song, DH β019, _Colored facial image restoration by similarity enhanced implicative fuzzy association memory‘, Indonesian Journal of Electrical Engineering and Computer Science (IJEECS), vol. 13, pp. 199-204.

57. Kimball, AB, Gladman, D & Gelfand, JM β008, _National Psoriasis Foundation clinical consensus on psoriasis comorbidities and recommendations for screening‘, Journal of the American Academy of Dermatology, vol. 58, no. 6, pp. 1031-1042.

58. Kimball, AB, Jacobson, C, Weiss, S, Vreeland, MG & Wu, Y 2005, _The psychosocial burden of psoriasis‘, American Journal of Clinical Dermatology, vol. 6, no. 6, pp. 383-392.

59. Le, NQK, Do, DT, Nguyen, NTK, Hung, TNK & Trang, NTT 2021, _Identification of gene expression signatures for psoriasis classification using machine learning techniques‘, Medicine in Omics, vol. 1, p. 100001.

60. Lin, GS, Lai, KT, Syu, JM, Lin, JY & Chai, SK β0β1, _Instance segmentation based on deep convolutional neural networks and transfer learning for unconstrained psoriasis skin images‘, Applied Sciences, vol. 11, no. 7, p.3155.

61. Liu, Z, Lv, X, Liu, K & Shi, S β010, _Study on SVM Compared with the other Text Classification Methods‘, Second International Workshop on Education Technology and Computer Science, China, pp.219-222.

62. Louppe, G β014, _Understanding random forests: from theory to practice‘, Cornell University Library, pp. 1–225.

63. Love, TJ, Qureshi, AA, Karlson, EW, Gelfand, JM & Choi, HK 2011, _Prevalence of the metabolic syndrome in psoriasis: results from the National Health and Nutrition Examination Survey, 2003–β006‘, Arch Dermatol, vol. 147, no. 4, pp. 419–424.

64. Lu Juan, Ed Kazmierczak, Jonathan H Manton & Rodney Sinclair β01β, _Automatic segmentation of scaling in β-D psoriasis skin images‘, IEEE Transactions on Medical Imaging, vol. γβ, no. 4, pp. 719-730.

65. Macatangay, JMA, Ave, T & Usatine, RP β017, _A Primary Morphological Classifier for Skin Lesion Images‘, VáclavSkalaUNION Agency, p. 10.

66. Muhaba, KA, Dese, K, Aga, TM, Zewdu, FT & Simegn, GL 2022, _Automatic skin disease diagnosis using deep learning from clinical image and patient information‘, Skin Health and Disease, vol. 2, no. 1, p.e81.

67. Nedoszytko, B, Sokołowska, WM, Ruckemann, DR, Roszkiewicz, J & Nowicki, RJ β014, ‗Chemokines and cytokines network in the pathogenesis of the inflammatory skin diseases: Atopic dermatitis, psoriasis and skin mastocytosis', Postepy Dermatol Alergol, vol. γ1, pp. 84-91.

68. Osuna, E, Freund, R & Girosi, F 1997, ‗Support Vector Machines: Training and Applications', A.I. Memo No. 160β, Artificial Intelligence Laboratory, MIT.

69. Pal, A, Chaturvedi, A, Garain, U, Chandra, A, Chatterjee, R & Senapati, S 2018. Severity assessment of psoriatic plaques using deep cnn based ordinal classification', In OR 2.0 Context-Aware Operating Theaters, Computer Assisted Robotic Endoscopy, Clinical Image-Based Procedures, and Skin Image Analysis: First International Workshop, OR 2.0, 5th International Workshop, CARE 2018, 7th International Workshop, CLIP, Third International Workshop, ISIC, Held in Conjunction with MICCAI, Granada, Spain, September 16 and 20, Proceedings, Springer International Publishing, vol. 5, pp. 252-259.

70. Pal, A, Garain, U, Chandra, A, Chatterjee, R & Senapati, S 2018, ‗Psoriasis skin biopsy image segmentation using Deep Convolutional Neural Network', Computer Methods and Programs in Biomedicine, vol. 159, pp. 59-69.

71. Panneerselvam, K & Nayudu, PP β0βγ, ‗Improved Golden Eagle Optimization Based CNN for Automatic Segmentation of Psoriasis Skin Images', Wireless Personal Communications, pp. 1-15.

72. Parisi, R & Symmons, DP β01γ, ‗Griffiths CE, *et al.* Global epidemiology ofpsoriasis: a systematic review of incidence and prevalence', The Journal of investigative dermatology, vol. 133, no. 2, pp. 377–385.

73. Patnaik, S, Singh Sidhu, M, Gehlot, Y, Sharma, B & Muthu, P 2018, ‗Automated Skin Disease Identification using Deep Learning Algorithm', Biomedical and Pharmacology Journal, vol. 11, no. γ, pp. 1429–1436.

74. Patwardhan, SV, Kaczvinsky, JR, Joa, JF & Canfield, D β01γ, ‗Auto-classification of acne lesions using multimodal imaging', Journal of Drugs in Dermatology: JDD, vol. 12, no. 7, pp. 746-756.

75. Pearce, DJ, Lucas, J & Wood, B β006, _Death from psoriasis: representative US data‘, The Journal of dermatological treatment, vol. 17, no. 5, pp. 302–303.

76. Perera, GK, Di Meglio, P & Nestle, FO β01β, _Psoriasis‘, Annual Review of Pathology, vol. 7, pp. 385–422.

77. Preeti K Suresh, Prameet Singh & Shailendra Saraf β01γ, _Novel topical drug carriers as a tool for treatment of psoriasis: Progress and advances‘, African Journal of Pharmacy and Pharmacology, vol. 7, pp. 138- 147.

78. Qin, Z, Liu, Z, Zhu, P & Xue, Y β0β0, _A GAN-based image synthesis method for skin lesion classification‘, Computer Methods and Programs in Biomedicine, vol. 195, p.105568.

79. Qiu, X, Sun, Z & Tan, T β005, _Global texture analysis of iris images for ethnic classification‘, In Advances in Biometrics: International Conference, ICB, Hong Kong, China, January 5-7, Proceedings, Springer Berlin Heidelberg, pp. 411-418.

80. Raj, R, Londhe, ND & Sonawane, R β0β1, _Automated psoriasis lesion segmentation from unconstrained environment using residual U-Net with transfer learning‘, Computer Methods and Programs in Biomedicine, vol. 206, p. 106123.

81. Raju, D, Shanmugasundaram, H & Sasikumar, R β0β1, _Fuzzy segmentation and black widow–based optimal SVM for skin disease classification‘, Medical & Biological Engineering & Computing, vol. 59, no. 10, pp. 2019-2035.

82. Randal Wickett, R & Marty O Visscher β006, _Structure and function of the epidermal barrier‘, American Journal of Infection Control, vol. 34, pp. S98-S110.

83. Rawat, AS, Rana, A, Kumar, A & Bagwari, A β018, _Application of Multi-Layer Artificial Neural Network in the DiagnosisSystem‘, A Systematic Review, vol. 7, pp. 138-42.

84. Raychaudhuri, SK, Maverakis, E & Raychaudhuri, SP 2014, _Diagnosis and classification of psoriasis‘, Autoimmunity reviews, vol. 13, no. 4–5, pp. 490–495.

85. Raychaudhuri, SK, Maverakis, E & Raychaudhuri, SP 2014, _Diagnosis and classification of psoriasis‘, Autoimmunity reviews, vol. 13, pp. 490-495.

86. Roslan, R, Jamil, N & Mahmud, R β011, _Skull stripping magnetic resonance images brain images: region growing versus mathematical morphology‘, International Journal of Computer Information Systems and Industrial Management Applications, vol. 3, pp. 150-8.

87. Roslan, RB, Razly, INM, Sabri, N & Ibrahim, Z β0β0, _Evaluation of psoriasis skin disease classification using convolutional neural network‘, IAES International Journal of Artificial Intelligence, vol. 9, no. 2, p. 349.

88. Roy, A, Pal, A & Garain, U β017, _JCLMM: A finite mixture model for clustering of circular-linear data and its application to psoriatic plaque segmentation. Pattern recognition, vol. 66, pp. 160-173.

89. Segal, M & Xiao, Y β011, _Multivariate Random Forests‘, Wiley Interdisciplinary Reviews: Data Mining and Knowledge Discovery, vol. 1, no. 1, pp. 80-87.

90. Shrivastava, VK, Londhe, ND, Sonawane, RS & Suri, JS 2015, _Exploring the color feature power for psoriasis risk stratification and classification: A data mining paradigm‘, Computers in Biology and Medicine, vol. 65, pp.54-68.

91. Shrivastava, VK, Londhe, ND, Sonawane, RS & Suri, JS β017, _A novel and robust Bayesian approach for segmentation of psoriasis lesions and its risk stratification‘, Computer Methods and Programs in Biomedicine, vol. 150, pp. 9-22.

92. Smith, KA & Gupta, JND β000, _Neural networks in business: techniques and applications for the operations research‘, Computers & Operations Research, vol. 27, pp. 1023–1044.

93. Smola, AJ 1996, _Regression estimation with support vector learning machines. Master‘s thesis, Technische Universit¨at M¨unchen.

94. Srivarre-Ratana, C, Konak, A & Smith, AE β00β, _Estimation of all-terminal network reliability using an arti6cial neural network‘, Computers & Operations Research, vol. 29, pp. 849–868.

95. Srivastava, N, Hinton, G, Krizhevsky, A, Sutskever, I & Salakhutdinov, R β014, ‗Dropout: a simple way to prevent neural networks from overfitting', The Journal of Machine Learning Research, vol. 15, no. 1, pp. 1929–1958.

96. Stitson, MO & Weston, JAE 1996, ‗Implementational issues of support vector machines', Technical Report CSD-TR-96-18, Computational Intelligence Group, Royal Holloway, University of London.

97. Tancharoen, D, Tantawiwat, P & Kovintavewat, P β019, ‗Medical imaging using automatic region of interest segmentation for psoriasis diagnosis', 34th International Technical Conference on Circuits/Systems, Computers and Communications (ITC-CSCC), pp. 1-4. IEEE.

98. Tancharoen, Datchakorn, Patinya Tantawiwat & Piya Kovintavewat β019, ‗Medical Imaging using Automatic Region of Interest Segmentation for Psoriasis Diagnosis', γ4th International Technical Conference on Circuits/Systems, Computers and Communications (ITC-CSCC), pp. 1-4. IEEE.

99. Tapak, L, Afshar, S, Afrasiabi, M, Ghasemi, MK & Alirezaei, P 2021, ‗Application of genetic algorithm-based support vector machine in identification of gene expression signatures for psoriasis classification: a hybrid model', BioMed Research International.Volume 2021, Article ID 5520710, pp.10

100. Traub, M & Marshall, K β007, ‗Psoriasis: Patho physiology, conventional, and alternative approaches to treatment', Alternative medicine review : a journal of clinical therapeutic, vol. 12, pp. 319-330.

101. Veropoulos, K, Cristianini, N & Campbell, C 1999, ‗The Application of Support Vector Machines to Medical Decision Support: A Case Study', ACAI99.

102. Wei, L, Gan, Q & Ji, T β018, ‗Skin Disease Recognition Method Based on Image Color and Texture Features', Computational and Mathematical Methods in Medicine, vol. 2018, pp. 1–1

103. Zheng, Q, Yang, M, Tian, X, Jiang, N & Wang, D β0β0, ‗A full stage data augmentation method in deep convolutional neural network for natural image classification', Discrete Dynamics in Nature and Society, vol. 2020, pp. 1-10. Article ID 4706576

104. Zheng, Q, Zhao, P, Li, Y, Wang, H & Yang, Y β0β1, _Spectrum interference-based two-level data augmentation method in deep learning for automatic modulation classification‘, Neural Computing and Applications, vol. 33, no. 13, pp.7723-7745.

105. Zhou, Y, Shi, C, Lai, B & Jimenez, G β019, _Contrast enhancement of medical images using a new version of the World CupOptimization algorithm‘, Quantitative Imaging in Medicine and Surgery, vol. 9, no. 9, p. 1528.

106. Zollino, M, Di Stefano, C, Zampino, G, Mastroiacovo, P, Wright, TJ, Sorge, G, Selicorni, A, Tenconi, R, Zappalà, A, Battaglia, A & Di Rocco, M β000, _Genotype–phenotype correlations and clinical diagnostic criteria in Wolf-Hirschhorn syndrome‘, American Journal of Medical Genetics, vol. 94, no. 3, pp.254-261.

LISTOF PUBLICATIONS

International Journal

1. **Mohan, S** & Kasthuri, N β0βγ, _Automatic Segmentation of Psoriasis Skin Images Using Adaptive Chimp Optimization Algorithm - Based CNN', Journal of Digital Imaging, vol. γ6, no. γ, pp. 11βγ-1136, **Impact Factor : 5.5.**

www.ingramcontent.com/pod-product-compliance
Lightning Source LLC
LaVergne TN
LVHW082347200926
848481LV00012B/3486
* 9 7 9 8 2 3 1 1 7 9 2 5 1 *